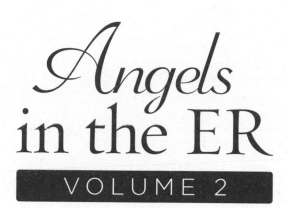

Angels in the ER

VOLUME 2

Robert D. Lesslie, MD

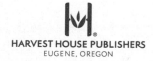

HARVEST HOUSE PUBLISHERS
EUGENE, OREGON

Cover design by Kyler Dougherty

Cover photo © gorodenkoff/Gettyimages

Published in association with the literary agency of The Steve Laube Agency, LLC, 24 W. Camelback Rd. A-635, Phoenix, Arizona 85013.

For bulk, special sales, or ministry purchases, please call 1-800-547-8979. Email: Customerservice@hhpbooks.com

> This book is not intended to take the place of sound professional medical advice. Neither the author nor the publisher assumes any liability for possible adverse consequences as a result of the information contained herein.
>
> Incidents described in this book are true. Names, circumstances, descriptions, and details have been changed to render individuals unidentifiable.

Angels in the ER Volume 2

Copyright © 2021 by Robert D. Lesslie, MD
Published by Harvest House Publishers
Eugene, Oregon 97408
www.harvesthousepublishers.com

ISBN 978-0-7369-8348-8 (pbk.)
ISBN 978-0-7369-8349-5 (eBook)

Library of Congress Control Number 2007052796.

Printed in the United States of America

22 23 24 25 26 27 28 29 / BP-RD / 10 9 8 7 6 5 4

To all those who have, are, or will work in an ER,
to my editor in chief—my wife, Barbara—
without whose help, like a sheep, I would have gone astray,
and to Carla Potts, Patricia Cline, Barry Benfield,
and Larry and Cathy Adams. You know who you are.

Contents

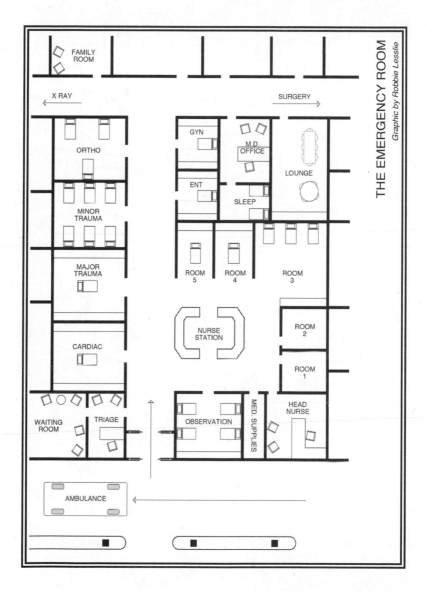

THE EMERGENCY ROOM

Graphic by Robbie Lesslie

FAMILY ROOM

X RAY

SURGERY

ORTHO

GYN

M.D. OFFICE

LOUNGE

MINOR TRAUMA

ENT

SLEEP

MAJOR TRAUMA

ROOM 5

ROOM 4

ROOM 3

CARDIAC

NURSE STATION

ROOM 2

ROOM 1

WAITING ROOM

TRIAGE

OBSERVATION

MED. SUPPLIES

HEAD NURSE

AMBULANCE

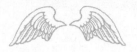

Angels Among Us

D r. Lesslie, have you *really* seen angels in the ER?"

Since my first collection of true stories from the ER was published more than 12 years ago, I've been asked that question a lot. It's been by readers from all over the world—and from every walk of life. Some are believers, some want to believe, and some have no belief. But it's never asked by someone who has worked in the ER. Never.

That's because those of us who have been privileged to work in the ER—those of us who have been able to care for people when their lives are slipping away, and to stand with loved ones in the moment of their greatest uncertainty, fear, or grief, and to rejoice when a life is saved—know that we are not alone. The distracting trappings of this world fall away, and we are able to glimpse unexplainable, even miraculous realities and ageless truths in this challenging and fiery crucible. Yes, there are angels. They pass through our lives every day—as coworkers, family members, or complete strangers. And sometimes in a form we can't touch, comprehend, or even begin to understand.

If you want to read about some of these inspirational encounters, you'll find them in these pages. And if you want to learn of some bizarre occurrences and outrageous patient behavior, you'll find that here was well. But most importantly, if you want to know what the presence of Jesus looks and feels like, spend some time with me in the ER and just ask Mike Brothers, or Tyler Anderson, or Stuart Gray. Better yet, simply read on.

Back from the Dead

All things human hang by a slender thread.

Ovid—43 BC–AD 17

Tyler Anderson was 33 years old when he died. Or almost died. If you ask him, he departed this earth for only a minute or so. If you ask me, it was an eternity.

Tuesday, 2:35 p.m.

Lori Davidson pushed an empty wheelchair through the Triage hallway, closely followed by Tyler, his wife, and two tow-headed young boys. Lori shook her head as she passed the nurses' station and muttered, "Hardheaded. Refused to let me wheel him into the ER. Insisted that he could walk fine on his own."

Tyler Anderson stood well over six feet, his muscled forearms sunburned and dusted with hay. His overalls were pulled from his shoulders and hung at his waist, and he clutched a bloody rag to the middle of his chest.

Lori led him down the hallway to Major Trauma, his young family silently ambling behind him.

"Hardworkin' man," Amy Connors, our unit secretary, said. "His family has farmed a couple of hundred acres out on Highway 5 for a lot of years. My husband and I run into him every

11

once in a while over at Farmer's Exchange. Good folks. Must be something serious to bring him to the ER, but he looks fine to me."

I had barely glanced at the man as he passed by. He didn't seem to be in any distress and had even managed a smile.

Lori walked up and dropped his clipboard on the countertop. "Blood pressure is good, and his pulse is normal. But he says he was working in his barn with one of his horses when it reared up and knocked him backwards. He fell and landed on some kind of rake, and one of the tines poked him in the chest, right below his sternum."

That got my attention, and my head jerked in the direction of Trauma.

"He's completely stable, Dr. Lesslie," Lori reassured me. "No shortness of breath, and his lungs sound great. It's his wife who insisted he come in to be checked. He'd rather be having all of his teeth pulled than be here right now."

I finished writing up the chart of the patient in room 4 and tossed it into the discharge basket, then picked up Tyler Anderson's chart.

Thirty-three-year-old male, normal blood pressure and heart rate, no medications, no allergies.

"Let's go see what's going on."

I closed the door of Major Trauma and walked over to the stretcher standing in the middle of the room. Tyler Anderson sat stiffly upright, with his arms folded across his chest and his legs dangling from the edge of the bed. He had the hospital gown Lori had given him on backwards, and it was opened in the front, straining to cover his burly chest. Behind him stood his wife and their two small sons. They looked to be close in age, probably seven or eight years old, and they pressed themselves tightly against their mother's legs.

"Mr. Anderson, I'm Dr. Lesslie. Tell me what happened today."

He fumbled with the gown, untied a single knot, and held it open. "I think I put this thing on backwards."

I nodded. He had, but it worked. His wound was in the front of his chest, and that's what I needed to see.

"Just right." I dropped his chart on the stretcher, stepped close to him, and gently examined the puncture wound in the pit of his stomach—just below the bottom of his sternum. A single drop of blood had dried over the small hole. There was another wound—a scratch, really—a few inches to the left.

"That's nothin', Doc," he said, following my eyes with his own. "This is the one Martha is so worried about." He pointed to the middle of his upper abdomen.

I continued to examine his chest and the puncture wound. "Tell me how this happened."

Tyler cleared his throat and sniffed loudly. "I was workin' in the barn, brushin' one of our new horses, when she spooked and reared up. I lost my balance and fell backwards. Landed on a brand-new rake we had just bought. Never been used. It was leanin' against a wall, and I must have grabbed it as I went down. It got under me and poked me in the chest. I must have fallen at an angle, 'cause only one of the tines got me. This other place is only a scratch."

I examined that area next, and he was right—this was a

superficial wound, the skin barely broken. It was the other one, the puncture wound just below his heart, that had me worried.

"I'm concerned about tetanus, Dr. Lesslie," his wife spoke up. "Even though that rake wasn't rusty or anything. We're not sure when he had his last booster."

"We'll take care of that," I told her. But I wasn't worried about him contracting tetanus. It's a common misconception that you get "lockjaw" from a rusty nail. That doesn't happen unless the nail happens to be on the ground in a farmyard or other outdoor area and is contaminated by the spores of the bacterium that causes the disease. Tyler had been working in a barn and would need a booster, but he wasn't going to get tetanus.

His lungs sounded good, and his heart tones were strong and regular. I didn't feel the "crunch" of any free air under his skin— an indication of a deeply penetrating injury. But I still didn't have an idea of the potential depth of this wound. And there were some pretty important structures not far below the surface.

"How long do you think the tines of this rake are?" I asked him.

Tyler glanced at his wife and then back to me. "Four, maybe five inches. Sharp and pointy, but like I said, clean as a whistle. I'm not sure how far that thing went in, but I landed on it pretty hard."

That was enough to concern me. "We'll get a chest X-ray to check on your lungs, and an EKG, just to be sure everything's okay with your heart. It won't take long."

I looked at the boys still pressed against their mother's legs. Two sets of large, brown eyes stared back at me.

"Doc, I'll be fine. If everything sounded okay to you, I'll just be headin' home and—"

His wife stepped to the bedside and put a hand on her husband's shoulder. "Tyler, just be still and let the doctor do what he needs to do. We want to be sure you're all right."

The door opened, and Sheila, one of our nurses, stuck her head in the room.

"Dr. Lesslie, we need you in Cardiac. Sixty-year-old woman with chest pain. Heart rate's 42."

I grabbed Tyler's clipboard and headed into the hallway. "We'll get those studies done as fast as we can."

Half an hour flew by, and the woman in Cardiac was stabilized—for the moment. She was in the middle of a heart attack but was responding well to a "clot buster." Her heart rate had improved—it was somewhere in the 60's—and she was already in the cath lab.

I was standing beside the counter in Cardiac, writing on the woman's chart, when Lori burst into the room.

"We need you stat in Trauma!"

The look on her face and the tone of her voice were all I needed. Without a word, I hurried behind her to Major Trauma. In the hallway, we passed one of our techs shepherding the Andersons' two small boys to the family room.

Sheila was feeling for a pulse over Tyler's left carotid artery and looked up at me with wide eyes, her face flushed. She shook her head.

I raced to the bedside and glanced at his chest X-ray hanging on the view box behind the stretcher. A fleeting look was all I could spare, but his lungs were fully inflated and his heart size was normal. Nothing unusual.

"What happened?"

Tyler Anderson's mouth was open, his facial muscles slack as he gasped for breath. His eyes were fixed on mine, but distant, unseeing. He was dying.

Sheila was saying something, but I didn't hear. The answer was screaming at me from right under her hands.

Tyler's face and neck were turning a mottled, dusky purple, and his neck veins—the jugulars on both sides—were bulging. A quick check of his lungs was normal—he was moving air. I placed my stethoscope over his heart and turned my head to the cardiac monitor. His heart rate was over a hundred, but...I couldn't hear anything. His heart tones had initially been strong, easily heard. And now silence. His heart was trying to beat, but nothing was happening.

"Give me a 20cc syringe and an 18-gauge needle. A long one."

I didn't have time to put on gloves—barely enough to take the Betadine and cotton gauze that Lori was handing me. Our eyes met. She knew what needed to happen.

The orange-colored disinfectant spilled down his abdomen as I wiped the area below his sternum.

"Tyler, I'm going to put a needle into your chest and into your heart. Hold as still as you can." He didn't respond. His dim and closing eyes now stared at the ceiling or somewhere beyond.

A quiet gasp penetrated the silence. I remembered that his wife was still in the room. From the corner of my eye, I could see Lori moving toward her and putting an arm around her shoulders.

I felt for the xiphoid—the bony tip of the sternum, and

placed the tip of the needle just below it, angled toward his head. The textbooks would tell you it needed to be attached to an electrode and the cardiac monitor so you could tell when you made contact with the heart.

We didn't have time for a textbook.

The needle punctured the skin and easily advanced through the soft tissues beneath. Then I felt it. The slightest resistance. It was his pericardium—the thin, fibrous lining around his heart. Normally, it contained only a few cc's of clear fluid, allowing the heart muscle to easily expand and contract within it. If I was right—and I prayed I was—the single tine from that rake had punctured the pericardium, causing blood to collect in the space between that lining and the heart itself. It didn't take much, and when a critical amount accumulated—especially quickly, not allowing time for accommodation or stretching—the heart would be increasingly squeezed, as if it were in a vise. It's called "tamponade," and it kills. The heart tries to beat but is unable, and blood backs up into the large veins of the body, especially in the neck—the jugulars.

I didn't hesitate, and slowly advanced the needle until I felt a "pop." There's no other way to describe it. I knew I had punctured his pericardium. I pulled back on the syringe and held my breath.

Nothing. No blood, no air. Nothing. I rotated the bevel of the needle and advanced it a fraction of an inch. Blood flashed back into the syringe—bright-red and beautiful. Five cc's, then ten, and then it stopped. A little more than two teaspoons. I pulled a little harder on the syringe, but nothing happened.

My heartbeat quickened, and I glanced at Lori. What now?

What else was there to do? I could crack his chest—make an incision between a couple of ribs, spread them apart, grab his heart, and cut open the pericardium. But the chances of him surviving that—

"Look." Lori nodded at Tyler.

I wasn't sure what she had noticed. His eyes were still closed and—

An arrow of hope pierced the gloomy and darkening cloud that surrounded his stretcher. The color of his face was improving—no longer the blotched purple of impending death. Right before our eyes, his skin was turning a light pink, and then a flushed, healthy red.

My eyes searched for his left jugular vein, trying to find it. It was no longer visible, but had sunk to its normal size. Blood was returning back into his heart, and it was beating.

"Good pulse over here," Lori said, her fingers spread over his right wrist.

Tyler gasped, and his eyes opened. He reached with one hand toward his chest, and I realized my needle was still inserted through his skin and into his pericardium. Lori handed me a piece of gauze, and I quickly withdrew the stylet and applied pressure over the needle's puncture site.

His color continued to improve, and he looked around the room. When he found his wife, he wordlessly reached out to her with an unsteady hand.

Lori took the blood-filled syringe, and we both stared at it. Just a little over two teaspoons of blood was all it had taken to turn things around for Tyler, to save his life.

"Good work, Dr. Lesslie," Lori said, with a smile of relief on her face. She noticed my hands were trembling, and our eyes met.

"Good work," she whispered.

The next morning, I went to the ICU to check on him. It was early, and Tyler was alone in the room. Martha must have still been home with the boys.

He lay quietly on the bed, looking out the large window as the scarlet-hued sunrise slowly chased away the darkness of a long night.

"Hey, Dr. Lesslie. Have a seat." He pointed to a chair pulled close to his bedside. The slow, steady bleep of his heart monitor was the only sound in the quiet room. An IV was taped to the back of his left wrist—the only other evidence that he was actually a patient in an intensive care unit. "The surgeon says I'm gonna be fine. I won't have to have any operation, and he won't need to poke me in my heart again." He chuckled and put his hand on his chest. "Whatever you did was all it took."

We talked for a few minutes about his injury and what we had done in the ER. And then we were quiet.

"You know, Doc, I was dead. Gone. I felt my life slippin' away, and there was nothin' I could do. And now I'm alive again. How many people does that happen to?"

He glanced out the window at the brightening sky and took a deep breath.

"The good Lord has given me another chance, a little more time. I don't know why, but He has. I think He has something for me to do, and I'm gonna find out what that is. Ya know, when you're lying in a hospital bed in the middle of the night, and it's all dark and quiet, you can't help but do some thinkin'. And lookin' back at things, I figure He's been trying to get my attention for a while now. I guess I've been busy with the farm and the cows and all."

He stopped and tapped the middle of his chest. "But if He meant for this to get my attention, it sure did. Things look a lot different this morning. I've got a better idea of what's really important and what I need to be doin'."

He paused and sighed. "I can't wait to see Martha and the boys."

Two days later, Tyler Anderson was released from the hospital. He and his wife had wanted to come through the ER on their way out and had stopped in front of the nurses' station.

Lori, Sheila, and I stood with them, and Amy Connors sat on the other side of the counter.

"Doc, you guys saved my life. I was gone and..." The words choked in his throat, and he looked away. He didn't need to say anything more.

We said our goodbyes, and Tyler promised to be more careful the next time he fell in the barn. They exited through the ambulance entrance, and as the automatic doors were beginning to shut, the younger boy turned.

His brown eyes were as large as ever, but this time, he was smiling. He waved as the doors whispered closed.

Tyler's words in the ICU had struck a chord, and I had once

again been reminded that life is a mystery and truly fragile. We're given only one, and we need to make it count. We need to find our work, and we need to see it through.

Not all of us get a second chance.

2

Say It Ain't So

Virginia Granger was on the warpath. And if you knew her, you'd know to get out of the way.

As the head nurse of the department, it was her responsibility to see that everything was handled properly—from supplies to equipment to personnel. It was the personnel part that was the most challenging.

She stormed out of her office, marched over to the nurses' station, and stood over our unit secretary.

"Amy, check and see what nurse is up on 4-B this morning, and get them on the phone. We transferred a patient up there last night, and they still have our stretcher and cardiac monitor. This is the third time that's happened in the past week."

4-B was one of the hospital's "med-surg" floors—a combination of medical admission patients such as those with pneumonia, dehydration, and other less critical problems, and those who needed postsurgical beds. It was usually well run and staffed with good nurses. It was unusual to have problems with them, but I knew better than to prod Virginia.

She was ex-military, and at age 62 was still as energetic and feisty as she must have been when she was 30. Ramrod straight and always dressed in an impeccably white uniform and starched white cap, she cast an imposing figure. Her jet-black eyes were piercing and quickly subdued the most egocentric of our medical staff. You didn't mess with Virginia, especially when she was riled.

Her hand began tapping the back of Amy's chair, and she pursed her bright-red lips.

Amy glanced up at me with widened eyes and a knowing grin. This might be good.

"Hey, Dora," she spoke into the receiver. "Can you talk with Ms. Granger?"

She held the phone over her shoulder, and Virginia grabbed it.

"Dora, we need to talk. I'm coming up."

She handed the phone back to Amy and headed down the hallway toward the back elevators.

"Whew," Amy whistled. "Wouldn't want to be on the receiving end of that."

"She'll cool off a little before she gets there," I said hopefully. "Dora Weathers is a good friend of hers."

She and Virginia had worked together in the ER for more than 20 years before Dora assumed the role of head nurse on 4-B, and Virginia took over the ER. The two units worked smoothly together, largely because of this friendship.

Half an hour later, Virginia was back in the department with the stretcher and monitor and was headed to her office. She caught my eye and motioned for me to follow.

"Pull that closed, will you, Dr. Lesslie," she told me, waving her hand at the door.

I did as instructed and sat down in front of her desk. This was a little unusual, and something was amiss. A moment of panic flitted through my brain as I wondered if I had transgressed in some fashion.

She rolled a pencil in her fingers and gazed at her hands. Finally, she took a deep breath, sighed, and looked up at me. "If you thought I was slipping, you'd tell me, wouldn't you?"

I was stunned and didn't know how to respond. Virginia slipping? Impossible.

"You mean mentally?" I asked her.

"Yes. If you saw that I was...that I was not as sharp..."

"Hold on a second, Virginia. What in the world are you talking about?"

She sighed again and leaned back in her chair.

"I was just upstairs talking with Dora Weathers about the problems we've been having with our patients going to 4-B. She and I go way back, and I know her like my sister. We're the same age, and Dora is one of the most capable nurses I've ever known. But this morning, there's something...She was having trouble focusing on what I was saying, and it scared me. It was a Dora that I didn't know, and I'm worried that if she..."

"You're worried that if she's having signs of some cognitive decline that you might be too?" I leaned forward in my chair and put both hands flat on her desk. "That's not happening, Virginia. There's nothing wrong with your mind. But tell me about Dora. Who's her doctor? And does she have any medical problems?"

Virginia stroked her chin and slowly nodded her head. "I'm not sure who her doctor is, but I know she's had some blood pressure issues for a while and been on medication. Don't know about any other medical conditions, but do you think she might have had a TIA or a small stroke? That might explain..."

"Why don't you ask her to come down to the department and let me take a look at her. If you're worried, let's just see what's going on."

She reached for her phone and started dialing. "I think she'd be fine with that, and it would make me feel better. Thanks."

Dora came to the ER during her lunch break, and I had a chance to talk with her in room 5. Virginia stood by the side of her stretcher and studied the two of us, her eyebrows closely knitted together. We talked for 15 minutes, and then Dora slowly got off the stretcher, stumbled a little, and walked toward the curtained opening.

"I'd better get back upstairs," she told us. "Thanks, Dr. Lesslie. And Virginia, let's talk later."

She left the room, and Virginia and I looked at each other.

Virginia had seen the stumble. "You see what I mean? Something's just not right."

I shared her concern. Something had changed with Dora—something over the past few weeks.

"Can you be sure she follows up with Dr. Kelsey?" I asked her. "He's a good doc and should be able to get a handle on this."

"You can be sure of that," she said while pulling a new paper sheet onto the stretcher. "And thanks for talking with her."

Stuff happens, and time passes quickly in the ER. I had forgotten about our encounter with Dora Weathers until a few weeks later when Virginia walked up to me.

"Well, Dora saw Dr. Kelsey, and he ordered some tests. Not sure what, but he didn't think she had any kind of dementia. And like us, he was worried about her balance. Apparently, she's been having more trouble and is more unsteady on her feet. I think she's been gaining weight too, but I'm not sure why. She's always been really active and walks a couple of miles every day after work. She and her husband, Ted. Maybe I should give him a call and see if he has any thoughts."

I signed the chart of the child in room 4 and slid it across the counter to Amy Connors.

"He needs a strep screen," I told her. Fever, sore throat, swollen tonsils, enlarged lymph nodes in his neck. This would be a straightforward diagnosis—unlike whatever issue was afflicting Dora Weathers.

"Just the two of them in the home?" I asked Virginia. "Dora and her husband?"

"No. They took in their 17-year-old granddaughter several months ago. The girl's parents divorced—a really ugly thing. She didn't want to live with either of them and asked if she could stay with Dora. Still in high school and having some problems, from what Dora tells me. That's a lot of stress that she really doesn't need. Yet, she wants to help, and I have to admire her for that."

That *would* be a lot of stress. You just never know the burdens other people are carrying, but she was confiding in Virginia, and that was positive.

"Ms. Granger! We need you upstairs on 4-B!" One of that unit's nurses had run down the hall and stopped in front of us.

Her face was red and her eyes wide-open. She looked from Virginia to me and said, "And we need you too, Dr Lesslie!"

We followed her down the hallway to the service elevators.

I pushed the "Up" button and asked, "What's going on? I didn't hear a code being called."

"It's not a code," she answered, mashing the button again. "It's nurse Dora. Something's wrong."

The elevator doors slid open, and we piled inside.

"What's going on with her?" I asked.

"I think she had a seizure." The young nurse was mumbling now, and tears welled in her eyes. "We got her flat on the floor, but she's just gazing up at the ceiling and won't say anything. Her blood pressure's low—70 over 40—and her heart rate is really slow. Only about 45."

Virginia looked at me. "You think this is a cardiac issue? She's never had anything wrong with her heart that I know of. Never smoked, no diabetes."

The door opened, and before I could answer, we were on our way toward the nurses' area.

A small crowd was gathered behind the counter, surrounding the prostrate body of Dora Weathers. She was breathing and moving one of her arms, but her color was a frightening pale green. Virginia cleared a path to her side and knelt on the floor.

"Dora! It's Virginia! Can you hear me?"

Dora's hand stopped moving and her eyes searched the crowd of faces—searching but not seeing.

I was on the other side and reached down to check her carotid pulse. Slow—really slow, but regular. Her skin was cool and damp, and her respirations were shallow.

"Let's get her on a stretcher and down to the ER," I told one of the staff. "And can somebody call the department and let them know we need Cardiac?"

We quickly had Dora loaded and on the way to the elevator. One of the floor nurses hurried alongside and handed me some papers.

"This is Dora's lab work—the studies done in Dr Kelsey's office. She and I were looking through it right before she collapsed."

"Thanks." I stuffed the papers into my lab coat pocket just as the elevator doors opened.

Lori Davidson was waiting for us in Cardiac.

"I've got the lab on the way and X-ray, if you need them," she told me.

"Great. We'll need a stat EKG, and give Respiratory a call. She's breathing on her own, but I don't know how much longer that's going to last. And we need an IV going wide open."

"Blood pressure's 72 over 40," one of the techs called out. "Pulse ox is 97 percent."

At least *that* was good news. A pulse ox of 97 percent indicated she was oxygenating her blood and perfusing vital organs.

"Heart rate's 38."

That wasn't good news. *Why was her heart rate so slow? We'd need to address that quickly if it didn't respond to some IV fluids. An EKG would help, but what was I treating?*

At the side of the stretcher, the EKG printed her tracing, and I picked it up. Slow rhythm, but everything else was normal. No evidence of any cardiac injury or electrical blockage. No answer here.

Labs were drawn, a portable chest X-ray had been done, and her IV was flowing smoothly. After half a liter, her color seemed a little better, but she remained confused and barely responsive. Virginia was glued to the head of the stretcher.

She stroked Dora's hair and spoke quietly to her. Her hand stopped moving, and she leaned closer to Dora's face, staring. With an index finger, she gently traced her right eyebrow.

"Strange," Virginia whispered. "I've never noticed that before."

"What?" I leaned forward, following her gaze to Dora's face, wondering what she was seeing.

She pointed to the outside half of Dora's eyebrow. "Here. Doesn't that look strange? It's the same on the other side."

I looked closer, still not seeing. And then I did. The outer third or so of each of Dora's eyebrows was hairless.

"That's something new," Virginia said. "I would have noticed it before, I'm sure."

A door cracked open somewhere in my mind. But only partially. I remember... It was something we learned in med school— some obscure piece of information. *What did this mean? It indicated something, but what?* It was in there somewhere, but I couldn't grab it.

"Here's her lab work," the tech said, handing me two pieces of paper.

"Thanks." I scanned the report for anything unusual, anything that jumped out at me, anything that might point us in some direction.

Her blood sugar was fine, as was her white count. She was a little anemic, but nothing dangerous. Interesting. Her sodium was low. Not dangerous, but still…

"Dr. Lesslie, this is Dora's husband, Ted." Virginia pointed me in the direction of the doorway. "And her granddaughter, Laney."

I stepped back from the stretcher and held out my hand.

"Mr. Weathers, your wife is stable right now," I told him. "And that's the good news. The challenge is trying to figure out what's going on with her, and I hope you can help."

He was a tall man, dressed in khakis and a blue, long-sleeved shirt. He stepped to the side of the stretcher and gently placed a hand on his wife's shoulder.

"I don't know…she's been quiet lately, and just not herself. But she hasn't complained of anything. Well, she complains about the house being cold. But it feels fine to me."

"Have a seat over here, Laney." Virginia shepherded the young woman to a stool in the corner of the room. She was tall also, and slender. Long, black hair flowed over her shoulders but couldn't quite hide the hollowed areas above her collarbone. *Too* slender.

Turning back to Ted Weathers, I asked, "What medications does she take? I think Virginia told me about her blood pressure, and she's on some medicine for that. But is she being treated for anything else? Any other problems?"

"She's on lisinopril for her blood pressure, but only a small dose. And she takes a bunch of vitamins—C and D and a B complex, I think. Maybe some biotin and cinnamon. And she's on her thyroid medicine."

"She's hypothyroid?" I asked.

"Yes. She's been on medication for 30, maybe 40 years. Pretty good dose, as I understand it—200 milligrams or micrograms. One of those. But it's always been controlled."

I reached for the lab work in my coat pocket and opened the crinkled pages. Dr. Kelsey had ordered a CBC, electrolytes, and a metabolic profile. That covered most of the important things. I scanned down the first page and then the second, looking for her thyroid studies. Not there. *Why would he not have ordered these?*

At the bottom of the second page was a note.

Lab error. T3, T4, TSH not performed. Please resend.

The date on the report was only a few days ago, so Kelsey wouldn't have had time to redraw and resend these thyroid studies.

"Virginia, call the lab to see if they can do a thyroid panel on the blood they have. If not, we need to restick her. Stat!"

Turning to Mr. Weathers, I asked, "Is she good about taking her medications? Ever miss her doses?"

"Dora?" He shook his head. "Never. She's the most organized woman I know. Keeps all her pills in a couple of those plastic weekly containers. You know, Monday, Tuesday, Wednesday. Makes me do the same thing. Like I said, she takes ten or twelve different things, but she keeps them organized and in the kitchen, right above the coffeepot."

That cracked door in my brain was opening, and some things were trying to fall into place. Confusion, cold intolerance, low blood pressure, mild anemia, low sodium. I reached down and pressed two fingers over her lower leg. There was edema present, but not "pitting edema," as you might see with heart failure. And then I remembered the eyebrows. The outer thirds were missing. That pathology lecture in med school that I had filed under "Interesting but will never use" surfaced, and I remembered the discussion about the eyebrows. The only thing I recalled it being associated with was a profound hypothyroidism. Something called *myxedema*. I had only seen one case of it in my career, and that was during my residency. Same picture as that of Dora Weathers. And the woman had died.

The lab tech burst into the room and thrust a report into my hand.

"The director wants you to see this! Now!"

It was Dora's thyroid studies. Her hormone levels were nonexistent. That confirmed my suspicions and explained all of her symptoms, but how could that be?

Turning to Mr. Weathers, I asked, "Are you sure she's been taking her thyroid medication? According to this report, she hasn't, and she's in trouble."

Ted shook his head and looked down at his wife. "She sets them out every couple of weeks and puts all her meds in three weekly containers. I don't see how she would have forgotten the thyroid. She's too careful about that."

It didn't make sense. I turned to Lori and ordered the medications that needed to be given quickly. They weren't routine, and I added, "If the pharmacy has any questions, ask them to give me a call."

The beeping of Dora's monitor was the only sound in the room. I looked across the stretcher into Virginia's eyes. She had a pensive look on her face, and her eyes were sharply focused behind me. I turned and followed her gaze.

Laney Weathers sat slouched on her stool, legs crossed and arms folded over her knees. Her vacant eyes scanned back and forth over the empty floor in front of her.

What had grabbed Virginia's attention. What was she seeing?

And then I noticed it. Her right hand trembled—barely perceptible, but she was shaking.

"Laney," I spoke quietly.

She looked up at me with wide eyes, then turned away.

Virginia was walking around the stretcher and stopped beside the young girl. She put a hand on one of Laney's shoulders, and their eyes met.

It all came together. Laney had fallen into the dangerous mindset of so many of our young people—especially young women. She was preoccupied with her weight and the pathologic obsession of being skinny. One of her friends had mentioned that thyroid medication would help you lose weight, and when she discovered there was some in her home, she started stealing Dora's medicine. It was easy to do. She found an over-the-counter medication that resembled the thyroid pill and switched them out of Dora's weekly containers. At first, it was only a few times a week. But when she started losing weight, it became an everyday occurrence. She didn't mind the rapid heartbeat or the increased nervousness. She didn't even mind the tremor in her hands, though that was getting worse of late. The biggest problem was that she didn't mind what it was doing to her grandmother. She was killing her.

Weeks passed, and one morning I remembered to ask Virginia about Dora.

"How is she doing? I heard she's coming back to work in a few days."

Virginia smiled and nodded. "It's really amazing. She's the old Dora—sharp as a tack and light on her feet. I can't keep up with her when we're out walking. And to think we almost lost her. It's all so hard to believe. If she had passed out at home by herself, or if she..."

"But she didn't," I interrupted. "And she's lucky to have you for a friend. But tell me about Laney. Where is she now?"

"Hmm," she muttered. "That's where Dora is a better person than I am. Laney is still living with Dora and Ted. Dora knew she didn't have anywhere else to go, and she wasn't about to send her out on her own. She's getting counseling now, and the last time I saw her, she'd gained some weight. I think she learned a hard lesson—one that she'll never forget." She paused. "She's lucky to have Dora. If anyone can keep her straight, it's her."

She took a deep breath and sighed.

"And...?" I asked.

Virginia looked at me over the top of her horn-rimmed glasses. "And yes. She's locking up her medication."

> *Grace is the very opposite of merit... Grace is not only undeserved favor, but it is favor, shown to the one who deserves the very opposite.*
>
> —Harry Ironside

Murphy's Law

There are a couple versions of what's commonly known as "Murphy's Law." In medicine, it seems the most appropriate wording is, *"Things will go wrong in any given situation, if you give them the chance."* I've seen it happen all too often. For Ben Whitley, well...he should change his name to Ben Murphy.

February—Friday, 6:30 p.m.

"Okay, let me guess."

Ben Whitley was lying on one of the stretchers in Minor Trauma. His left pant leg had been cut off, and a bloody bandage was covering his thigh. I picked up a corner of the gauze and gently raised it, exposing a five-inch laceration that started just above his kneecap. Its edges were ragged, and it pointed down and out.

"Chain saw," I said.

The 45-year-old man looked up at me and grinned. "How'd you know that?"

I tossed the bandages into a kick bucket at the end of the stretcher and walked over to the supply cabinet. "I've seen a few," I answered. "That angle, that depth, chewed-up edges. That's a chain saw signature."

"You're right, Doc. I was out cuttin' firewood, and it was gettin' dark. I had just told myself I needed to quit before somethin' happened, and then it did. Foot slipped, I guess."

Lori Davidson walked into the room, followed by Denton Roberts. He and his paramedic partner had just brought a "chest pain" patient in by ambulance and got him settled in Cardiac.

Lori took a look at the exposed wound and said, "I'll get a suture tray set up. Anything special?"

"Yeah," Denton said, stepping around her to the head of the stretcher. "This is Ben Whitley, Doc, and he's a friend of mine. Try to save his leg if you can."

He winked at Whitley, who was now looking at me with wide eyes, head cocked to one side.

Lori shook her head as she opened the suture kit and spread its contents on a sterile towel.

With a serious tone, I said, "I'll do what I can."

"What?" Ben looked first at me, then at Denton.

"Don't worry," Denton laughed. "You're in good hands. But what were you doing out this late cutting firewood? It was getting dark at five o'clock."

"I knew better. Time just got away from me, and it just happened."

I slipped on a pair of sterile gloves and sat on a stool beside his stretcher. Lori pushed the tray up beside me, and I reached for the syringe of lidocaine.

"This is going to sting a little," I warned him and began anesthetizing the jagged edges of the gaping wound. Once the medicine took effect, I probed the area, looking for pieces of bark and making sure the large tendon in his thigh was intact.

"Looks good here," I told him. "You're lucky. Sometimes these can really be a problem. You okay so far?"

I glanced up at him. He was intently watching everything I was doing and nodded his head.

"I'm fine," he told me.

I glanced at the pocket of his long-sleeved hunting shirt and saw an opened pack of Marlboro's.

"We need to talk about those," I said, motioning my head in the direction of the cigarettes.

"You tell him, Doc," Denton interjected. "I've been on him ever since high school, trying to get him to quit. I've even tried to get him to ride along with us one evening and see some of our COPDers. Just can't get through his thick skull."

"Denton's right, you know," I said to Ben. "That's probably the most important thing you can do about your health right now. It's tough to stop, but there's nothing good that comes from smoking those things."

Ben nodded silently and stared at his thigh.

"And while we're here, why don't you tell Dr. Lesslie about your belly pain," Denton said. "It's time you did something about that."

Whitley seemed relieved to change the subject. He looked up at me and began describing the pain he had been having for the past year. I listened while continuing to trim away dead tissue and piece together the edges of his laceration. When he paused, I asked a few questions about the timing of the pain, its quality, and things that made it better or worse. It sounded like his gallbladder, and while more common in women his age, men were not immune to gallstones or inflammation of this organ.

It took about an hour to put him back together, and during that time we discussed what I thought was going on with his belly pain and how we should approach things. The first step would be to get him in with his family physician, but when he told me he had none, I asked Lori to have our unit secretary line him up for an ultrasound in the next few days.

"Doc, just so you know, I don't have any insurance," Ben said. "Is that going to cost a lot?"

"Doesn't matter what it costs," Denton told him. "You need to get this figured out, and I know a couple of us will be glad to chip in if you need it."

His radio squawked, startling the three of us. "Medic 1, respond."

"That's me," Denton said, grabbing his radio and heading for the door. "Gotta go."

Ten minutes later, Ben was on his way out of the ER. His left thigh was heavily bandaged, and his pants were missing the left leg. Not an unusual scene in our department.

He waved the order sheet for the ultrasound in his hand and turned to me. "Thanks, Doc, and thanks for this."

"They'll send me the results," I responded, "and as soon as I hear, I'll let you know."

Amy Connors, our unit secretary, looked up as I walked into the department. Three days had passed since Ben Whitley had been in the ER.

"Got something for you," she said, sliding a single-page report across the counter. "Ben Whitley's ultrasound."

"Good. I'm glad he got it done."

I set my briefcase on the floor, picked up the paper, and quickly scanned it.

"Well, I guess that's it. Looks like Ben is going to need his gallbladder taken care of."

The report was straightforward, indicating that he had several gallstones and a thickened and inflamed gallbladder wall. This was the cause of his pain, and he would most likely need surgery.

"Can you get Walt Summers on the phone for me?" I asked Amy. He was one of the general surgeons in town and a friend.

"Sure," she answered. "Give me a sec."

I walked back to our office, grabbed my lab coat, and headed back to the nurses' station. Amy held out the receiver and said, "Summers."

I told Walt about Ben, his symptoms, the ultrasound report, and the issue of his insurance status. It complicated things, but Walt didn't hesitate.

"We'll take care of that. Just have him call the office, and we'll see what we need to do. I'll let you know, Robert. And thanks."

It was a good start for the day. Straightforward diagnosis and plan of treatment. We would be able to help Ben Whitley and make his life a little better.

Two days later, Walt Summers walked through the department. I was standing at the nurses' station finishing up a chart, and he walked over.

"Saw your Mr. Whitley in the office yesterday. He's a good guy, and I'm in agreement with your thoughts. He needs to have his gallbladder out."

I wanted to quote the well-worn surgical adage that "a chance to cut is a chance to cure," but decided against it. While not always true, it was so in this case.

"I got some blood work in the office," Walt continued. "His blood sugar is up a little, as was his cholesterol. He doesn't take any medicine, and he told me he hasn't seen a doctor in years. We did an EKG too, and it was a little off. Just some nonspecific stuff, but with his smoking history and cholesterol, I've asked Winston Abrams to take a look at him."

Winston was a cardiologist on our staff—young, smart, and he took care of his patients. It would be necessary, but I couldn't help but sigh when I considered the cost of all this. And we hadn't even gotten to his surgery.

"Thanks for seeing him, Walt. Keep me posted on what's going on. He *is* a good guy."

"Code Blue! Cardiology unit!"

The announcement of a "Code Blue" was the hospital's urgent signal of an emergency, usually a cardiac or respiratory arrest. The call came over the hospital intercom and was repeated. One of the ER doctors on duty needed to respond to the code—something bad happening in the Cardiology suite. I was gloved and suturing a patient in Minor Trauma and was about to strip off my gloves when Brad Hayes appeared in the doorway. He was one of my partners and had come on duty about an hour earlier.

"I'll get it," he told me. "Keep doing what you're doing." He disappeared down the hallway, followed by one of our nurses.

Forty-five minutes later, I was standing at the nurses' station.

Brad walked up and grabbed the chart of the next patient to be seen.

"Everything okay in Cardiology?" I asked him. The Cardiology suite was where the heart caths were done in the hospital. There were always a few cardiologists present, and they could handle most emergencies that might arise. But they were always thankful for our help.

"Yeah, well...sort of."

Brad shook his head and continued. "Winston Abrams and his partner were doing a cath on a young guy. Apparently, he had a couple of significant blockages that needed fixing, and they were able to put a stent in one of them. When they started with the next vessel, it spasmed, and he went into full arrest. No cardiac activity for more than half an hour, but we got him back. He's a tough bird and still heavily sedated. Just have to wait and see if his brain was affected. Couldn't fix the blockage and had to stop the procedure, so he still has a 90 percent occlusion in one of his coronary arteries. I guess that will have to wait. Bad luck, for sure."

"Did you happen to get a name?" I asked him.

"I think I heard Whitley, but don't quote me."

Ben had seen Winston Abrams in his office. After a failed stress test, Abrams advised a heart catheterization to evaluate and define any significant blockages in his cardiac vessels. Without that information, any planned gallbladder surgery could be dangerous. The procedure had been scheduled, and now the Code Blue. He was 45 years old—a young man. Way too young to be having this kind of problem.

At the end of my shift, I went upstairs to the ICU to find Ben and check on him. He was resting quietly in one of the cubicles but opened his eyes as I walked into the room. His wife was sitting in a chair by his bedside.

"Hi, I'm Dr. Lesslie," I addressed her.

"He's the one who started all of this," Ben chided me, but with a smile on his face and a twinkle in his eye. How could that be possible? The man had been clinically dead for 30 minutes and was lying in a bed in the ICU.

"Thanks, Dr. Lesslie," his wife said. "I'm Sue Whitley. Ben told me about how you've tried to help him."

"I didn't expect this," I stammered. "It was supposed to be straightforward, simple."

"It happens, Doc," Ben said. "But take a look at this."

He raised his right hand and reached for the sheet. His fingers trembled, and his arm drifted aimlessly. He dropped it to the bed and raised his other hand.

"That's getting better," he told me. "Seems like I had a little stroke while I was out, and it affected my right arm and hand. Getting better though."

He raised the sheet with his left hand, exposing his left thigh.

"Remember this?" he asked, pointing at the healing scar just above his knee.

The wound was healing well and looked fine.

"This looks great," I said, gently palpating the edges of the laceration. "Who put this back together?"

"Some yahoo in the ER. I guess I got lucky."

We talked some more about what had happened and what the next steps would be.

"Oh, and it looks like I'm now a diabetic," he added as I was stepping to the doorway. "My blood sugar has gone sky high, and they started me on insulin. Don't know where that came from. No family history or anything. We'll just have to deal with it."

I didn't say anything, but I couldn't help but wonder what else could go wrong.

Two days later I found out what that "else" could be.

Walt Summers was in the department examining a seven-year-old boy who had what I thought was appendicitis. I stood beside him while he gently probed the child's abdomen. The boy grimaced when Walt felt his right lower quadrant.

"Hmm...I think you're right."

He explained his findings to the anxious parents and his recommendations for surgery. We left the room, and as we walked down the hallway he said, "I guess you heard about Ben Whitley."

"I know about the cardiac arrest, and that he's been in the ICU," I answered. "Seems to be getting better, but boy...what bad luck."

"It didn't stop there," he said, shaking his head. "One of my partners was on call last night and had to come in about two in the morning. Whitley was having severe leg pain, and the nurses were worried about a blood clot. They were right. Looks like a clot developed where the catheter was placed in his groin, and he lost blood flow for a while. That cleared on its own somehow, but when Jake saw him, he had already developed a compartment syndrome. Happened fast, and he was in a lot of pain."

"A compartment syndrome? How did that..." I was struggling to put all of this together.

The two most common areas of the body where this syndrome can occur are in the forearm and the lower leg. There are "compartments" in these areas—several groups of muscles, nerves, and blood vessels that are bounded by fibrous tissue. Any significant swelling within these compartments can squeeze the blood vessels, depriving the affected muscles of blood flow. It can happen after a significant contusion or anything that causes blood or fluid to collect in that space—like a clot. If not quickly corrected, the muscle will die. Forever. And the pain is terrible.

"I know." Walt shook his head. "Jake had to do a fasciotomy in the ICU, and we'll just have to see how he does. Pain's better, but we won't know about the muscles for a few days. Maybe longer."

I grimaced at the word *fasciotomy*. It was a barbaric but limb-saving treatment—one that I had done several times in the ER. It was simple, requiring only a surgical blade and the will to slice into the compromised compartment. You have to go deep enough to penetrate the fascia, freeing the underlying muscle and restoring blood flow. *Filet* is the way it's described. And that's accurate. The endangered muscle protrudes through the wound—frequently eight to twelve inches long—and is left like that, covered with sterile dressings, then later repaired. You just hope and pray that the muscle survives.

The muscles in Ben's leg partially survived. He lost strength in that leg—something that rehab would help, but he would never return to where he was before.

Several months passed. One early Saturday morning, Denton Roberts and his partner were in the ER having delivered two patients from an MVA to Minor Trauma. It was raining, and this would be one of many fender benders that would be treated in the department.

He walked past me at the nurses' station, and I thought of Ben Whitley.

"How's your buddy Ben?" I asked him.

Denton stopped and looked at me. He shook his head and said, "You know, Doc, he beats all. You know about everything that happened to him—way too much for any one person. Heck, just one or two of those things—the stroke or the compartment syndrome—would be enough to get most people really down. But not Ben. He's getting around the best he can with a cane and trying to do some work for some folks. Says he can't sit still and needs to be doing something."

"Hope he's not doing any more chain saw work," I chuckled. "But at the end of all of that, he still has a bad gallbladder and a vessel in his heart that needs to be fixed. That has to be weighing on him."

"It might be," Denton nodded. "But you couldn't tell it by talking to him. He's got the same grin on his face and the same twinkle in his eye. It's still Ben Whitley, after all that he's had to go through."

How does someone do that? How can one man handle such a load without giving up?

Denton must have been thinking the same thing.

"I don't know how I'd deal with what he's had to deal with. It all happened so fast. But you know, Doc, he has a good family and a wife who loves him. And his faith is as strong as an oak tree. I think that's it—his faith. And I think that's what he would tell you."

Murphy's Law. This was never Ben Murphy. This is Ben Whitley.

> And we boast in the hope of the glory of God. Not only so, but we also glory in our sufferings, because we know that suffering produces perseverance; perseverance, character; and character, hope. And hope does not put us to shame (Romans 5:2-5).

4

I Don't Like Spiders or Snakes

Some people are natural targets for a practical joke. And then there's Sharon Brothers, otherwise known as "Crash."

I should probably start by admitting that early on in my life I was asked to take the following oath: *I solemnly swear that I am up to no good.*

To this day, I don't think I've broken that promise. Crash is one of the reasons why.

February—a dark and...freezing night.

The ER was quiet. Finally. It was 3:00 a.m., and you'd hope that would be the case. EMS 3 had brought in a 20-year-old who had slipped—with the aid of a few adult beverages—on a patch of ice and bruised his tailbone. He had been evaluated, treated, and was on the way out the door. The department was empty.

Crash Brothers and her partner on EMS 3, Clarence Chapmen, were sitting with us at the nurses' station, talking about the cold weather, the runs they had made during the day, and the hopes of a quiet rest of the night.

Crash leaned back in her chair and folded her hands behind her head.

"It's so cold that Grannie's teeth are chattering...in the glass," she quipped.

"What?" Jeff Ryan had walked up to the counter. "What do you know about flashers? Oh, wait a minute, didn't you..."

"Hold on right there, buddy," Crash stopped him. "That's just about enough."

"Crash," I leaned close. "I didn't know you..."

"And that's enough out of you, Dr. Lesslie."

Jeff Ryan was the nurse on duty tonight. He was big, burly, and intimidating to the uninitiated. But to those who knew him, he had a huge heart—one that matched his abilities as an ER nurse. If it was out there, he had seen it. And if it wandered into our ER, he had treated it. Perhaps his best attribute was that he was my willing and capable partner when it came to playing jokes on unsuspecting people. Crash was one such person, and when combined with a quiet moment in the ER, well...anything could happen.

Jeff walked around the counter and stood beside Crash. In his hand was a clipboard, and he held it out in front of the EMT.

"Did you leave this back in Minor Trauma with the guy you just brought in?"

She looked at the board and shook her head. "No, I've got my stuff here."

As hoped, she took it in her hand and flipped over the top sheet.

"Ahhhhh!!!!"

Crash jumped out of her chair and sent her chart, the clipboard, and her dignity flying. Jeff had carefully placed a rubber snake under the top sheet of paper, and Crash had done what she was supposed to do. The rest was...well, everyone at the nurses' station was laughing—except Crash.

Flushed, she finally recovered enough to point a finger at Jeff and say, "You think that's funny? I almost wet myself."

Her fear of snakes was legendary, matched only by that of spiders. One afternoon, Jeff had come across a picture of a hairy tarantula, and he slipped it inside the menu of a local eating establishment.

"Crash, we're going to order takeout," he told her, holding out the menu. "You want something?"

You'd think that after a dozen or so years, she would know better. But no.

"Well, sure. Let me take a look."

She took the menu and opened it.

"Ahhhhh!!!"

Amy Connors, our unit secretary this cold February evening and a person known to appreciate some levity, looked over at Crash.

"Tell Dr. Lesslie what you told us about the psych patient you picked up earlier."

Amy leaned back in her chair and waited.

"Oh boy, that was a doozy!" Crash dropped into her chair again, but not before casting a reproachful glance in Jeff's direction. "We had a call over on Strait Street, something about a man wandering in his front yard in his underwear. Dead of winter, mind you! Turns out he had stopped his medication from the mental health center a couple of weeks ago and was out of control, preaching about the end times. He kept talking about 'Possum lips' and how we all had better get ready."

"Possum lips?" I asked, trying to figure this one out. She was known to scramble her words a little. She had once given me a report about a young man with "abominable pain." It turned out to be appendicitis, and I should have known.

"Yes, he kept talking about the end of the world and possum lips."

It finally dawned on me. "You mean the Apocalypse?"

"Yeah, the possum lips," she answered, not missing a beat. "The end times—and we all better be gettin' ready. It was all we could do to get him in the ambulance."

Amy shook her head and winked at me. She wasn't finished.

"Crash, tell us again about your neighbor back when you were growing up and that Sunday school song."

"How'd you remember that?" she asked, leaning back in her chair again and grabbing both of its arms. She slowly began to rock and started her story.

"I was 14 or 15 years old, and it was one of those things—like you've always thought one way for most of your life, and then you find out you've been wrong the whole time. We had a neighbor back then, an old farmer named Jethro Klein. He was a good guy and always brought us pears and persimmons when they were in season. And it didn't surprise me any when I'd hear the junior choir singing about 'Jesus loves old man Klein.' I know Jesus loves everybody, and Mr. Klein was a good man, so it didn't surprise me. I mentioned that to my momma one day, and she said,

'What? Old man Klein? Honey, the words of that song go, 'Jesus loves all mankind.' You could'a knocked me over with a feather. All those years and I thought it was 'old man Klein.''

I shook my head, wondering in amazement. Now it was my turn.

"Crash, you know Freddy Gaskins, don't you?"

"Freddy?" she answered, smiling. "Sure. We go way back. He's been a highway patrolman for...for as long as I can remember. Why?"

"Well," I began, "he was in here the other night and was telling us about an accident on Highway 21."

"That's a bad stretch of road," she nodded, pursing her lips. "Specially right there where it goes from four lanes to two. People don't pay attention and bam! We've responded to a bunch of MVA's out there."

"That's exactly where this happened," I nodded, suppressing a grin. She was helping me tell this story.

"Anyway, Freddy responded to a call—a 10-50—out on 21, right where you're talking about. Single-car accident. It was dusk, and the light was fading fast. At first, he couldn't see any damaged vehicles or any sign of an accident. Then, off to the right of the highway, he saw a station wagon with its front end jammed into a big oak tree. Smoke was coming from under the hood, and he pulled over, grabbed his flashlight, and went straight to the car to see if there were any victims. The car was empty, and he started looking around the scene."

"Bet some drunk ran off the road and then took off runnin','" Crash interjected knowingly. "Happens all the time."

"No," I continued. "Freddy saw a group of people 20 or 30 yards away, all sitting together under another big oak. He walked over and saw it was a family—a mother and father and two young kids, a boy and a girl, about ten or eleven. The father had a scratch on his forehead, but nobody seemed really hurt. They were all just sitting there, real quiet. Well, Freddy walks over and takes out his notepad.

"'Anybody want to tell me what happened here?' he asked them.

"Nobody said a word. They just stared off into space.

"'Okay, sir,' he said to the father. 'I need to know what happened. What caused this accident?'

"Nothing. They just stayed silent. Not a peep."

"Seen that happen too," Crash interrupted. "People won't talk. Don't want to admit nothin'."

"Well, nobody was saying a word, and Freddy was starting to lose his patience. All of a sudden, he noticed some movement off to his left. He scanned the area with his flashlight, and when he came to the station wagon, he saw a monkey sitting on the hood."

"A monkey?" Crash burst out.

"Shh," Jeff Ryan quieted her. "This is a true story."

"Yes, a monkey," I resumed. "It was sitting on the car waving its arms in the air. Freddy kept staring at it, and the monkey started jumping up and down and pointing to itself. Finally, Freddy got it.

"'Oh, so *you* know what happened here?' he asked.

"The monkey started nodding his head.

"'Well, then, let's see. What was *he* doing?' Freddy directed the beam of his flashlight on the father.

"The monkey raised his little finger and thumb, shaking it back and forth, with his thumb pointing to his mouth. Freddy had to think about this for a moment, but then he figured it out.

"'So this guy was drinking?'

"The monkey nodded excitedly.

"'Okay, this is starting to make some sense,' Freddy said while jotting some notes onto his pad. 'And what about her?'

"This time he pointed to the mother. The monkey raised both arms in the air and made flapping motions with his hands.

"'Hmm...Oh, I get it! She was nagging him.'

"The monkey once again jumped up and down, nodding his head.

"'Now we're getting somewhere,' Freddy said.

"A few more scribbled notes, and then he pointed to the children. 'And just what were they doing?'

"The monkey started punching the air in front of him.

"'They were fighting!'

"The monkey's head went up and down.

"'Well, that just about explains it.' He made some more notes, emphatically put a period at the end of the statement, and closed the pad.

"He was walking back to his patrol car when he stopped and looked once more at the monkey.

"'Just for my information, what were *you* doing?'

"The monkey looked at him for a moment. Then he raised

both arms, made fists in the air, and moved them in a circular motion.

"'Oh, now I see,' Freddy said. 'You were driving.'

"The monkey nodded his head."

"Now that's a bunch of junk," Crash exploded.

"What?" Jerry said from behind her. "I told you this was a true story."

"Nope," she said, folding her arms across her chest and shaking her head. "Everybody knows that monkeys can't drive."

There were scattered chuckles, and I just shook my head.

"Ahhhhh!!!"

A scream, loud enough to wake the dead, startled everyone in the department.

Seconds earlier, Jeff had caught my eye and winked. Out of his pocket, he had taken a three-inch plastic spider attached to a piece of fishing line. From behind Crash, he had dangled this in front of her face, eliciting the bloodcurdling response. Her arms flew wide, and her legs went up in the air.

"Dagnab it! I *did* wet my pants this time!"

Suddenly, her radio squawked, commanding everyone's attention.

"EMS 3, respond code 3 to a 10-50."

It was an MVA, and they needed to go fast. Crash and Clarence bolted out of their chairs and headed for the entrance.

"It better not be out on Highway 21," she hollered as the ambulance doors opened, inviting in a blast of freezing air. "And Jeff, just you wait!'

They were gone, and we sat in silence looking at each other.

Crash Brothers. What would we do without her?

Mirth is the sweet wine of human life. It should be offered sparkling with zestful life unto God.
                    —Henry Ward Beecher

5

A Country Road

The path to our destination is not always a straight one.
We go down the wrong road, we get lost, we turn back.
Maybe it doesn't matter which road we embark on.
Maybe what matters is that we embark.

—Barbara Hall

The nature of the ER is such that we have a number of physicians who appear out of nowhere looking for work. It might be for a few weeks or months, or maybe for more permanent employment. Frequently, their training or work history make it obvious that they're just not a fit for our department. More frequently though, we—Virginia Granger and I—just have a gut-level feeling that something's not quite right. Maybe it's eyes that won't meet ours or a troubling sense that what we're hearing just doesn't add up. But every once in a while, someone will walk into the ER that we immediately know needs to be there. And we make a place for them.

6:55 a.m.

"That's it? Just the kid in 3?"

Moss MacLeod snapped shut his battered briefcase and

looked at me with sleep-deprived eyes. He was the overnight doc, and I was his relief.

"That's it, Robert," he answered. "His blood work should be finished when he gets back from ultrasound, but regardless, he's got a hot appendix. Dr. Boyle is on for surgery, and you know he won't slice a Thanksgiving turkey without a scan. Just waiting on that. We've already notified the OR, so things should move pretty quickly."

I chuckled and shook my head. "You're right about Boyle— unfortunately. Now, go home and get some rest."

Virginia Granger, our 62-year-old head nurse, walked up beside me as the ambulance entrance doors closed behind Moss.

"Not sure how long that's going to last," she said quietly.

"What? You mean Moss?" I searched those piercing eyes hidden behind her 1960s black, horn-rimmed bifocals, hoping for some clue as to her comment. "You think he's overqualified to be working here with all of his experience?"

"No, not that," Virginia answered. She pursed her lips, bright red with recently applied lipstick. "He's carrying some baggage. I just don't know what."

She knew more about his "baggage" than I did, just as she did for everyone who worked in the department. But I knew about his prior ER experience and qualifications. They were impressive. Moss MacLeod was 44 years old and a native of Louisiana. When I had remarked that MacLeod was not a typical name for that particular part of the country, Moss was quick to inform me of his family's ancestry, only four generations removed from the clan's origins on the Isle of Skye. My wife and I had visited there with our children, and Moss and I talked about Castle Dunvegan and the incredible vistas gained from a hike into the Quiraing.

"I think Clan Leslie hails from the Aberdeen area," he had said. And he was right. We had that Scottish heritage in common— that and the fact that we were both bagpipers.

Moss had completed his undergraduate work at LSU, and then medical school there as well. He met his wife while an emergency medicine resident at Grady in Atlanta—a program that baptized you with fire and molded you within its blazing furnace. Most came out as refined gold, but not a few were reduced to a pile of ashes. Moss was golden, and he and his wife moved to Baltimore, where he was on the faculty of Johns Hopkins—another demanding and prestigious institution. After a few years, his wife insisted on moving south, and they settled just outside Athens, Georgia. He worked there in the ER of Athens Regional Medical Center.

A few years later, his wife died, the circumstances of which were vague and not completely known, even to Virginia Granger. There followed a three-year gap in his work experience, until he showed up at the nurses' station one day, wanting to speak with me. We needed some help, and after talking with him and reviewing his educational background and experience, I had offered him a job in the ER. He accepted.

That was five months ago, and he had fit into the department as if he had been with us five years. He was quiet at times, but always engaged, always approachable. The patients and our staff loved him. It had only taken two months for him to make a name for himself, to begin carving his legend as an ER hero. At 3 a.m. on a cold winter's night, he had managed to safely deliver twins in the front seat of a pickup truck in the ER parking lot. And a few weeks later, he saved the life of the son of one of our nurses. The five-year-old had collapsed in the midst of an allergic reaction—his airway had closed off, and he had no pulse. Moss had scooped the boy in his arms and raced into the Cardiac room. He got him breathing again and reestablished his heartbeat. Today he's completely normal.

Now this from Virginia. The emotional baggage of losing his wife was significant, but what other things did she know about? I didn't want to lose him and wondered if I should be worried.

I turned to say something to her, but she had disappeared into her office and closed the door behind her.

Moss was sweating and short of breath. He glanced at his stopwatch and slowed to a fast walk.

Just under 42 minutes. Better.

He was on Fishing Creek Road and at the halfway point of his six-mile run—marked by a weathered and battered mailbox, probably dented by the multiple passings of teenagers with baseball bats. He would never understand why that would be a favorite pastime for 18-year-olds who lived out in the country.

On cue, he heard the fierce barking of a large pit bull, barreling toward him down a graveled driveway. The dog was snarling, its eyes squinting with malicious intent.

Calmly, Moss stopped, turned toward the threatening canine, and said, "Satan, it's only me."

The pit bull's countenance immediately changed, and his hard-charging attack morphed into a tail-wagging, torso-wriggling saunter. The dog sidled up to Moss, rubbing his neck against the man's thigh.

Moss had caught a glimpse of the dog's name tag a few weeks earlier and used it, along with a practiced—though cautious—unfrightened demeanor to make friends with the dog. It had all worked, and they were now fast buddies. He rubbed the dog's ears and chest.

"Good boy," he soothed the beast. He reached into his pants pocket and retrieved a small treat, adding reinforcement for the friendship and a little insurance. "Here you go. You go back home, and I'll be on my way."

Satan wagged his tail a few more times, turned, and trotted back up the driveway.

Whew! That dog could do some damage if he put his mind to it.

Moss glanced at his stopwatch again, reversed direction, and headed back toward town. He was still out in the country, not too far from the Chester County line, and there were few cars even at this time of day—the middle of the afternoon. He liked it this way.

His mind wandered to the ER schedule for the remainder of the week. He had a couple of nights coming up, and then he was off for the weekend. For most people, that would be cause for rejoicing. For Moss, it was just more empty time he would have to fill. He slowed and cocked his head in the direction of an unexpected sound—an unfamiliar wailing. It was a siren, the likes of which he had never heard.

A long straightaway of asphalt veered to his right, disappearing into a cluster of cedar trees.

The noise was getting louder. Moss stopped and stepped well out of the road, just as an ambulance careened into view, barreling straight at him. Lights flashing and siren blaring, the driver occupied the middle of the road, but not without difficulty. He was weaving from side to side, the vehicle being obviously unstable at this high rate of speed. Moss moved further into the shoulder, distancing himself as much as possible.

This was an ancient, elongated automobile, dating from the 1950s or '60s, and resembling more of a repainted hearse than an ambulance or rescue vehicle. Its warning light was perched on top, with the light making a slow, sweeping arc, like a lighthouse. And the siren…It was a loud, ear-splitting *whoop—whoop—whoop*.

The passenger was waving frantically at Moss, motioning him to get out of the way. There was no place for him to go unless he jumped the rusted, barbed-wire fence that was pressing into the back of his legs.

The ambulance sped by, and for an instant, the driver and Moss locked eyes. He slowly stepped back into the highway and took a deep breath. Then another noise caused him to freeze where he stood. A loud and sudden screeching as the vehicle braked, swerved to the right side of the road, and kicked up a cloud of dust and gravel. The driver slammed the vehicle into reverse, and they were heading back toward Moss again, swerving dangerously from side to side.

Moss jumped back onto the grassy shoulder as the ambulance came to a stop right beside him.

The passenger rolled down his window and stuck his head into the afternoon heat.

"Aren't you one of those ER doctors over at Rock Hill General?"

It was hard to fluster Moss MacLeod, but this was an encounter he hadn't expected. "Yeah, I'm Dr. MacLeod. You guys need some help?"

"Come on, get in!" The passenger jumped out and opened the backseat door, motioning Moss to get in. He was wearing navy pants and a white, long-sleeved shirt—buttoned at the top—with some kind of an emblem on the pocket that Moss couldn't read and didn't recognize. "I'm Sam Tinker, and this is Jerry Wilson," he said, pointing to his partner. "We're with the Chester County Rescue Squad, and we're respondin' to a call about a mile or two from here."

Moss climbed awkwardly into the rear-facing jump seat, cramped against what served as a stretcher, though it might have been one of the original gurneys from the town in California that bore that name and where gurneys originated.

Sam twisted around in his seat and smiled at Moss. "We don't have much equipment, as you can see. And we're not really with the Rescue Squad. More like *volunteer responders,* ya know. We try to help out when there's an emergency and nobody else is nearby."

"Like today," Jerry chimed in. "There's a big wreck out on the interstate—a couple of tractor trailers, I think—and just about every paramedic unit from Chester and York counties are tied up over there. Our scanner picked up this call, and we live only a few minutes from here, so we thought we'd take it. And then I saw you standin' beside the road, and I said, 'Sam, that's one of the ER docs over in Rock Hill.' Imagine that. Out here in the middle of nowhere."

"What kind of emergency are we responding to?" Moss asked, not a little uneasy.

"It's Clyde Turnstill," Sam answered. "He has a small shop on his place, and his wife called 911 with some kinda chest injury."

"Anything else?" Moss asked. "Is he awake? Breathing?"

Sam shook his head. "She didn't say. I guess we won't know 'til we get there."

The ambulance slowed and turned onto a rutted, dirt driveway. An arrow on a rusted sign pointed them toward *Clyde's Welding and Metal Works.*

"Clyde's a good guy," Jerry said. "Hardworkin' fella, with a wife and three kids. I hope he's okay."

The road twisted through some honeysuckle-entwined pine trees and then opened into a small clearing. Off to the right was a low-lying building, its garage doors open and revealing several machines, barrels, and tools of every description.

"That's his shop," Sam said, pointing out his window to the building.

"And there's Clyde and May Lee," Jerry added, bringing the vehicle to a stop in the middle of the clearing.

A 40-something-year-old man was lying on his back halfway

between the shop and the house. He wasn't moving, and his wife knelt by his side. One of her hands rested on his chest, and the other gently stroked his forehead. She looked up at the ambulance with terror-stricken eyes.

"Please help him!" she pleaded.

Two teenage girls and a younger boy stood behind her, their faces pale, eyes staring at the three men who scrambled from the rescue vehicle.

Moss was the first to reach Clyde, and he took a knee opposite the man's wife.

"I'm Dr. MacLeod," he told the two of them. "Tell me what happened."

Sam and Jerry rushed up, stood behind Moss, and leaned forward with hands on knees.

Clyde was awake and calm, and his color was good. Moss checked his carotid pulse and waited for the man's response.

"I...my..." he mumbled.

"I was in the house when I heard a loud noise," May Lee interrupted. "Sounded like a gunshot, and I tore out here to see what was going on. Clyde was inflating a tire when it blew, and something hit him in his back. That's all I know. He won't move. Just lies there."

Clyde stared into the blue sky and nodded. Moss noted that he was moving his arms and legs—relieved that his spinal cord seemed to be intact—and his chest rose and fell with each respiration.

A little afraid of the answer, he turned to Sam and asked, "Do you have a stethoscope?"

Sam jumped up and headed toward the ambulance. "Yeah! Give me a second."

"Let's take a look," Moss said, reaching over Clyde's torso to help him roll over.

"No!" Clyde's eyes were wide, and his right hand flew up and grabbed one of Moss's arms. "No!"

Moss backed off and studied the man's eyes.

"Want us to help, Doc?" Sam volunteered.

"No," Moss said, beginning to understand the situation. "What kind of emergency equipment do you have, Jerry?" He was afraid of the answer.

"Sam, go get the kit," Jerry instructed his partner. "Not much, Doc. Like we said, we only respond to calls if the EMS people need extra help. We're not first responders and all that."

Sam ran to the ambulance and back, carrying a worn and dirty zippered duffel bag. He dropped the kit beside Moss and opened it.

It was what Moss feared. A pair of scissors, a couple rolls of tape, some gauze, rumpled candy bar wrappers, and wait...

"Hand me that angiocath," he instructed Sam.

"The what?" Sam peered into the bag, shaking his head.

"The big needle," Jerry said, reaching into the bag and pulling out a 14-gauge IV needle and catheter, still in its plastic wrapping. "Don't know how old this is, Doc. One of the paramedics in Rock Hill gave us some stuff a few years ago when it went out of date. Should have thrown it away, I guess. But you never know."

Moss grabbed the needle and studied its plastic wrapping. He didn't care about the expiration date—only that it was still sterile.

He looked into the bag again. "Hand me some of those Beta-dine pads and some gauze. And I'll need some gloves." They wouldn't be for him but for Clyde. If Moss was right about what was going on, he would need at least part of one. "Is that Vaseline? I'll need that too, and some string."

Sam reached into the bag and picked up the half-empty jar of Vaseline. "Yeah, we use this to grease the stretcher when it starts to squeak a little. Smells better than WD 40. But I don't know about any string." He fumbled through the kit's contents and pulled out a small spool of umbilical tape—the kind used to tie off the umbilical cord after a delivery.

Moss barely suppressed a chuckle as an image of Jerry and Sam delivering a baby flashed into his mind.

He turned to Clyde while Sam and Jerry were getting the supplies together.

"Clyde, I need to roll you over and take a look at your back."

The man's eyes widened, and he shook his head.

"I know," Moss reassured him. "I know you don't want to move, but I need to see your back and try to help you."

"Clyde, do as he says," May Lee said, with a new edge of firmness in her voice, barely disguising her fear.

He looked up into Moss's face and slowly nodded.

"Sam, I want you to help me roll him over," Moss instructed. "And Jerry, put a bunch of Vaseline on a piece of gauze and have some tape ready."

"Gotcha, Doc."

"And hand me a knife," Moss added.

The two girls gasped, and Clyde looked into Moss's eyes.

"Sorry," Moss said. "It's for your shirt. I need to get it off, and I don't want you moving your arms around."

Jerry handed Moss a Swiss pocketknife, and the ER doctor deftly rendered the piece of clothing into shop rags. A quick inspection didn't reveal any injury to the front of Clyde's chest.

"Okay, Sam, I want you to gently roll him over, but as fast as you can without hurting him. Got that?"

"Sure, Doc."

"Gently," Moss repeated

Sam reached over Clyde and put one hand behind his right shoulder and the other on his right hip. He turned him quickly but smoothly. Clyde grimaced and muttered a muffled moan. That was the only sound, until the hissing. Just below Clyde's right shoulder blade was a one-inch puncture wound. There was only a little blood, but with each breath, air bubbled through the torn flesh.

"Hand me that gauze!" Moss ordered.

Jerry gave him the makeshift bandage, and Moss pressed it to the sucking gash.

"Let's roll him back over, Sam. I think this will close it off, and the pressure of the ground on his back will help."

The two men returned Clyde to his previous position, and the man sighed with relief.

"We've closed off that hole, Clyde. So you can relax a little."

Clyde had instinctively known what was wrong—a sucking chest wound that was allowing air to move into his chest cavity with each breath and be trapped there, creating pressure against his lung. The technical term was *tension pneumothorax,* and uncorrected, it would kill him. No wonder he was adamant about staying on his back and not exposing the hole to the open air.

"Jerry, do you have a radio? We need to get a helicopter here ASAP and get him to the trauma center in Charlotte. No time for land travel—not with the traffic this time of day."

Jerry stroked his chin. "We have a radio, Doc, but it's not much good. I might be able to reach dispatch and get them to call the trauma center. I can try that."

Moss turned and glared at the man. "I don't need you to *try,* Jerry. I need you to get it done."

Jerry struggled from his kneeling position and ran to the ambulance.

Now Moss had to fix the pneumothorax—the air that was trapped between Clyde's inner chest wall and his lung. He couldn't tell how big it was, but it had to be evacuated. There was a hole in his lung too. But that would have to be fixed in the operating room, if they could get him there.

"Sam, hand me that Betadine and angio...IV needle."

Moss turned again to Clyde. "We've got a dressing on that wound, but we need to put a needle in your chest and get rid of any air that's collecting between your lung and chest wall. I'm sorry I don't have anything to numb your skin with, and this might hurt a little. But we've got to do it."

Clyde's expression didn't change, and he nodded. May Lee pulled her children close and turned them around, trying to shield them from what was about to happen.

Moss looked over at her. "Ma'am, you may want to..."

"We're not movin'." The tone of her voice left no room for discussion, and there was no time.

Moss turned back to the task before him and opened a half dozen Betadine packets and wiped a hand-sized area over the side of Clyde's right chest. He opened the angiocath and inspected it one more time. No rust. No discoloration of the plastic catheter that was on the outside of the needle itself. The needle would be withdrawn, but it was this catheter that would remain inside his chest.

Satisfied, he looked into the man's face and said, "Okay, Clyde, just hold still. This is going to be uncomfortable, but then it will be over."

Jerry ran up behind them, waving an oversized and battered radio in the air. "I got through to dispatch, and a helicopter should be here in about 20 minutes!"

Moss nodded but didn't say anything. He was carefully palpating a couple of Clyde's ribs, locating the right spot to insert the needle.

"Here we go," he said quietly.

The needle pierced Clyde's skin, and he grunted but didn't move. Moss advanced it carefully, waiting for the palpable "pop" that would indicate its passing through the lining of his chest cavity and into the collection of air between that lining and Clyde's lung. Moss hoped it was air and not a large collection of blood. That would be another problem.

He felt the "pop" and then heard the loud and welcomed hiss of escaping air. May Lee gasped and put a hand to her mouth. Sam muttered, "Good Lord!" and Jerry dropped the radio to the ground.

Moss withdrew the metal needle, leaving the catheter in place, and dropped it onto the pile of Betadine swabs. He secured the catheter with his thumb and long finger and used his index finger as a stopper, preventing any further air from entering Clyde's chest.

"Be careful with that," he told Sam, pointing at the needle. "And hand me that glove and tape—and those scissors."

Sam reached into the bag, scrounged around, and held the supplies in two outstretched hands, waiting for further instructions.

"Anything else?" he asked.

"Not yet." Moss needed another hand, maybe two. "Sam, pick out a finger on that glove and cut it off—about two inches long."

"Cut off the..." Sam mumbled, staring at the surgical glove.

"Cut off one of those fingers," Jerry echoed loudly. "Here, hand it to me."

Sam handed his partner the glove and scissors and watched as Jerry neatly severed one of the fingers, then handed it to Moss.

"This do?"

"Perfect," Moss said. He took the latex finger and quickly slid it over the end of the catheter, snugging it to Clyde's chest. No hissing this time, and Moss relaxed a little.

"Now that umbilical tape. About five inches of it."

Jerry still held the scissors. He picked up the roll of tape and cut the requested length.

Moss used it to secure the glove over the catheter, then used bandage tape to attach this makeshift device to Clyde's chest. When he was satisfied with his handiwork, he leaned over, his ear only an inch or two from the catheter, and listened. Nothing. No leak. No bubbling around the small plastic tubing. And no hissing.

He let out a loud sigh and turned to Jerry one more time.

"Hand me those scissors."

Jerry dropped them into Moss's hand and watched open-mouthed as the ER doctor held the floppy rubber digit and snipped the end off. More hissing as air escaped through the new opening. Then just as suddenly as it started, silence. The finger collapsed upon itself, forming an airtight barrier.

"Air can get out," Moss explained, looking down at Clyde. "But it can't get back in. This will act like a one-way valve and will prevent that collection of air getting bigger and pressing on your lungs and heart. It buys us time but doesn't fix the main problem."

May Lee leaned close. "Is he going to be..."

She stopped and looked over the treeline behind Moss. They all heard it and followed her gaze. It was the rhythmic thumping of a helicopter, getting louder and closer with each passing second.

"I'll move the ambulance," Sam hollered, running toward the vehicle. "Give them some more space."

Moss turned back to Clyde. "How do you feel? I hope that didn't hurt too much."

"It hurt some, but like you said, it was over pretty quick. And I can breathe better."

Clyde took a deep breath and air hissed through the glove's fingertip.

"Probably need to take shallower breaths," Moss told him. "Just what you think you need."

The helicopter had landed, and the three crew members raced toward them. One carried a large medical box and the other two a lightweight metal stretcher. They wore bright-red jumpsuits, with the name of the trauma center clearly visible front and back. The paramedic carrying the box dropped it beside Clyde and put a hand on Moss's shoulder.

"You can back off now," the medic told him. "We'll take over."

Moss didn't move. He looked into the young man's face and said, "Let me tell you what we've got and what you need to do."

The two other crew members were kneeling on the other side of Clyde, one checking his blood pressure and the other using a stethoscope to check his breath sounds.

"We heard it was some kind of chest wound," one of them said. "Here, Chuck, help me roll him over."

Chuck had one hand in the air when Moss grabbed it, his face red and getting redder.

"Don't move him." The words sliced through the air, leaving no room for questioning or negotiation. "I'm Dr. MacLeod, an ER doctor in Rock Hill, and this is my patient. Understood? I'll tell you what happened to him, what I did, and what you're going and not going to do."

The three helicopter crew members stiffened and stared at each other.

"Understood?"

Moss hadn't let go of Chuck's hand, and when he did, the paramedic backed away.

"Okay, doctor," the lead paramedic muttered. "Tell us what's going on so we can get him loaded and on the way."

Moss described Clyde's injury, what he thought was going on, and what he had done to get things stabilized.

"The Vaseline and gauze should keep the wound of his back closed, as long as you don't mess with it. And this," he pointed to the catheter taped to Clyde's right chest, "will keep him from developing a tension pneumothorax. Got it?"

The paramedics glanced sideways at each other and nodded.

Moss stood and squared himself in front of the lead paramedic. "Now let me make this clear. Clyde is alive and breathing, and if you guys get him in the chopper and start messing with stuff, he's going to get into trouble. I know there's no room, or I'd be on board with you. But if anything happens to this man, you'll wish you never landed here."

The paramedic backed away, and when he answered, his voice was trembling. "Understood."

Within minutes, they had him on their stretcher and safely in the helicopter. May Lee walked over to Moss and hugged him.

"Thanks, doctor. I...I don't know what else to say."

"That's plenty, ma'am. Now you and your kids need to get up to Charlotte. Do you know how to get to the trauma center?"

He gave them directions as they piled into an old Suburban. Dust filled the clearing as they disappeared from sight.

Sam was cleaning up the used supplies, and Jerry grabbed their medical kit and walked over to Moss.

"Wow, that was somethin', Doc. Never seen anything like it. Hey, how about me and Sam driving you back over to Rock Hill or wherever you live? That's the least we can do."

Moss took a deep breath and smiled at the men.

"You know, I appreciate that. But I think I probably need to do some more running. Sort of work off all the excitement."

"I understand that," Jerry nodded.

Moss shook hands with the two men and watched as they climbed into their ambulance. Jerry made a wide, sweeping turn in the clearing and stopped beside him. He rolled down the window and said, "I hope we see each other again, maybe over in the ER. But not out here again." He chuckled and they drove away.

The dust settled, and the rattling, rumbling motor of the ambulance faded until it finally disappeared. Quiet.

Moss heaved a sigh and gazed up into the cloudless sky. He felt a familiar hand on his shoulder, and then heard that deep, soothing voice.

"You did a good job, Moss. I'm proud of you."

It was the voice of his grandfather.

He turned around...and was alone.

Major Trauma at Charlotte Regional Medical Center was frenetic—barely organized chaos—with a dozen members of the trauma team bustling about, honing in on their assigned duties. The helicopter crew had moments ago brought Clyde Turnstill into the large, open room and transferred him to the trauma bed. The lead paramedic reported what they had found at the scene, including a middle-aged man in running shorts, who claimed to be an ER doctor in Rock Hill.

"Crazy as a coot, if you ask me," the paramedic added. Yet, none of them had touched the bandage on Clyde's back or the catheter in his side. He had remained stable—remarkable, considering the nature and severity of his injury.

The trauma team captain was examining Clyde's chest, listening to his breath sounds.

"Well, I'll be. Would you look at this." He pointed to the tape on Clyde's right chest, and the improvised chest tube. The rubber valve still fluttered out with each breath, then collapsed again. "Mr. Turnstill, whoever did this knew what he was doing. He saved your life."

"I know who did it."

The words sliced through the air, dripping with disgust and loathing.

Every eye turned toward the third-year emergency medicine resident, and they waited in stunned silence for her to say something else.

Her face flushed, and her eyes narrowed when she spat out, "It's my father."

She turned and walked out of the room.

> *It is easier to tell the toiler*
> *How best he can carry his pack*
> *But no one can rate a burden's weight*
> *Until it has been on his back.*
>
> —Ella Wheeler Wilcox

6

Broken

The ER—9:35 p.m.

Wˢ need some help out here!"
One of the hospital's security guards was standing in the ambulance entrance, pointing frantically out into the parking lot.

"Somebody's having a baby!"

Jeff Ryan raced past me into the night and toward a Volkswagen camper. It was pulled up on a curb, and its side door was flung open.

Lori Davidson followed, pushing a stretcher. "Amy's calling Labor and Delivery," she shouted over her shoulder.

This was not an uncommon occurrence. Young women in labor would frequently present to the ER—or the ER parking lot—triggering a cascade of activity. Usually, there was time to get them upstairs to the more controlled environs of L and D, where the child could be safely delivered. Not this time.

Waiting in the entrance, I heard the cry of a newborn, protesting its sudden arrival into a strange and foreign world. Jeff quickly moved the mother to our stretcher, Lori held the blanketed newborn boy in her arms, and they rushed into the department.

Two nurses from Labor and Delivery were waiting at the nurses' station.

"We'll take her upstairs," one of them said to Lori. Then looking at me, "Can you check out the child until one of the pediatricians gets here?"

"Sure," I answered. "Lori, let's take him to Trauma."

"He'll be okay, right?"

The voice was quiet, trembling. My attention had been focused on the baby, and now I looked down at the mother.

"He's going to be fine," I told her. "We'll get him upstairs to you as quickly as we can."

Lori was walking past the stretcher, and the woman reached out to touch her child. Her bare arm was completely covered with tattoos, and my eyes were drawn to the inside of her elbow. Angry, red lines squirmed snakelike beneath the visible skin not covered by a multi-colored dragon. Some were obviously infected and draining.

"We gotta go," the L and D nurse said, whisking the woman down the hallway.

"Dr. Lesslie, we've got a problem here."

Jeff was calling out to me from Trauma, and I hurried into the room.

Lori and Jeff were on each side of the stretcher. My first glimpse of the boy in the hallway had been brief, but he appeared to be full-term and active. Now he was seizing.

"When did this start?" I asked, stepping over to the baby.

Lori was in the process of staring an IV and said, "Just now.

When we were getting him cleaned off, he seemed to be sweating a lot, and then he stiffened—then he started this."

He was in the midst of a generalized seizure, and we had to act fast.

"The back of that VW van was a mess," Jeff told us. "Filthy mattress, a bunch of dirty clothes, and half a dozen empty pizza boxes. She must have been living in that thing. And I can't be sure—it was dark, and we were moving fast—but I thought I saw needles and drug stuff scattered around."

It all came together. The red streaks on her arm were infected needle tracks, and now the newborn's seizure. This child was withdrawing from some medication that his mother was abusing. Probably an opioid. Possibly heroin. This was a fast onset for withdrawal symptoms, but it all depended on when the mother last used.

We worked feverishly to stabilize the baby and quickly had the seizures under control. But the care of this child would be beyond the capabilities of Rock Hill General, and I asked Lori to call EMS and arrange for transport to Charlotte Memorial.

"And see if Amy can get the ER doctor on duty on the phone. I need to let them know about this baby."

"Hey, Doc," the security guard called to me from down the hallway. "Whoever was driving that VW just took off. He's gone."

I shook my head.

Fifteen minutes later, Jeff was still in Trauma, cleaning up. I walked in and looked around. The room was quiet, as was Jeff. Too quiet.

"You okay?" I asked him.

"No, I'm not," he said angrily. "And I know *you're* not. How can someone bring a child into the world like that? The back of that van was filthy, and to be pregnant and using drugs...If that baby dies..."

I felt the same burning anger. Jeff and I both had young children, and we both knew how precious each one of them was. This was impossible to comprehend. And the anger was impossible to quench.

"You're right, Jeff. How can you understand or make any sense of this?"

"Dr. Lesslie." Shannon Meadows, a senior staff member with DSS, stood in the doorway. "I need to talk with you about the newborn you just sent to Charlotte."

Two hours later, one of the ER residents at Charlotte Memorial called me. She gave me an update on our baby—"Baby X." He had no name yet. We were right about the heroin, and right about our treatment. Baby X was stable—no more seizures—but still in serious condition.

"He should be fine," the resident told me. "But he'll be here for a while. And I'm sure you've gotten in touch with protective services."

"They just left," I told her. "They're upset and have gotten the police involved."

"I think we're all upset," she responded. "Anyway, good work with this child. Just wanted you to know where things stood."

I hung up the phone and turned to Jeff. He was standing nearby and heard the conversation.

"That's good news about the baby," he said. "Meadows told me their people would press for complete separation. That's the best thing for the child, but he's going to grow up without a mother. What a mess."

It was hard to have any sympathy for the mother, yet she was still the mother. She would soon realize that her child was gone—separated by her own irresponsible choices. How would she ever be able to forgive herself? And the boy—how would he be able to forgive a mother who cared more for herself than for her child?

3:00 a.m.

We had cleared out the department, and Amy was back in the lounge getting something to eat. I sat alone at the nurses' station, reading one of her *People* magazines, catching up on our culture's important matters, things I may have missed.

The Triage door opened, and Moss MacLeod ambled into the department. He was wearing running shoes, camouflage hunting pants, and a Carolina Panthers pullover.

The camo pants reminded me of one of his first shifts in the ER and when Amy had asked him about his name.

"Your name's not really Moss, is it? There has to be a story there." She was never one to be shy.

He explained that his given name was Carson, after his grandfather—a country doctor of more than 50 years. His own father had left when young Moss was nine years old, never to be seen again. His grandfather raised him, taking him along on house or farm calls, teaching him what he was able to absorb about life and death and disease and healing. And he taught him how to hunt turkey.

His grandfather would say, "If you want to be a turkey hunter, you have to learn how to call them in, make sure you're downwind, and sit still as a rock."

Moss paid attention, especially to the "sitting still as a rock" part. So still that one morning his grandfather remarked that he was so quiet and motionless, moss would grow on him.

The nickname stuck, and he had been "Moss" ever since.

On another occasion, Moss shared with me some of those medical experiences he had with his grandfather. Though his grandfather was long dead, Moss sometimes felt his presence—a warm, reassuring awareness—almost something tangible.

"Hard to explain," he had said. "Sometimes it's almost like he's pointing me toward something I should do or away from something that will lead to trouble. Usually, I just get a sense that he approves of me, and that...that means a lot."

"Looks like you've got things under control," Moss said, pulling up a chair and collapsing into it.

"Amy would say you just cursed us, but yes, we're finally under control."

"Busy shift?" he asked.

I wondered why he was here at 3:00 in the morning and what might be on his mind. It probably wasn't good. He was not just checking to see how busy we were.

"Busy up until about 2," I told him. "Just like always." Then I told him about the precipitous parking lot delivery and the newborn's withdrawal symptoms.

"Sounds like an opioid withdrawal," Moss observed. "There's a lot of heroin on the street."

"That's what we thought. Got a call about an hour or so ago from the ER at Charlotte Memorial. I talked with one of the ER residents...Lexi something. Didn't catch her last name. It *was* heroin, and the baby is doing okay."

"Lexi?" he repeated.

"Yeah. I heard the secretary call out to a Lexi, telling her that the ER in Rock Hill was on the phone, but I didn't catch her last name."

"Lexi MacLeod," he said slowly, his voice dropping.

"Mac...Leod," I fumbled.

"Yes. My daughter."

Moss and his wife had one child, Lexi. From as early as they could remember, she had wanted to become a physician and follow in her father's footsteps. After her undergraduate education at the University of Georgia, she attended the medical school at LSU, just as Moss had done. During any breaks, she would spend time with her father in the ER, shadowing him as he took care of patients in the Athens ER.

"She wanted to see everything," Moss told me. "Wanted to learn everything. I showed her some of the tricks I had picked up, and some of the things my grandfather had taught me. He had an uncanny way of seeing into a person's mind and figuring out the nature of their real problem—what had brought them into his office. And his skills with a physical examination... Well, he of course practiced in the days before CT scans or ultrasounds—even had a hard time getting an X-ray done. He knew his anatomy, and he trusted his hands. But he used to tell me that a good physician could usually make the correct diagnosis just by listening to his patient. Give them enough time, and they would tell *you* the diagnosis. The physical exam just confirmed it. I think Lexi understood that, even though that's not what they were being taught in med school. Tests and imaging. You know how that works, Robert."

Moss's eyes had brightened as he told me of these times with his daughter. Then his mood darkened.

"I think Lexi was in her second or third year of medical school. She had just spent a little time with us over Christmas and was back in class. We had lost some of our staff in the ER, and I was working a lot of shifts just to keep things covered. Too many. Looking back, I'm not sure when it started, or how I could have missed it."

He sighed, and his shoulders slumped. "But I missed something. My wife, Aubrey, is not a complainer, and I should have paid attention. She was starting to have some headaches—tension, she thought. From the holidays. I was busy and always exhausted when I got home from work. I think I may have told her to take some Tylenol and get some rest or something. I just didn't pay attention. Then one morning—it was a Tuesday at 9:18—she called the ER and told me that her headache was back and that it was the worst she had ever had. Finally, a light came on and I told her to call 911 and get to the hospital. I was frantic and

and bolted out of the ER. When I got to the house, her car was in the driveway, and there was no ambulance. I found her...I found her on the kitchen floor with the phone still in her hand. She was gone."

He fell silent. I didn't know what to say. What *could* I say?

"As I'm sure you've already guessed, Aubrey had a massive intracranial bleed and died instantly. An autopsy found a ruptured berry aneurysm—one that had been leaking for a few weeks. The headaches she was having were warning signs—signs I should have picked up on. She could have had that aneurysm clipped. If I had a woman her age in the ER and she told me..."

His words faded to a husky whisper.

"Moss," I said, putting a hand on his shoulder. "I don't know..."

My own words trailed off. I didn't know what to say to this man. What an impossibly heavy burden to be carrying. What an unbearable grief.

He took a deep breath and straightened in his chair.

"Lexi has always blamed me for that. She blames me for the death of her mother. And she's right. If I had paid attention, if I had only listened, Aubrey...Aubrey would be alive today."

"Moss..."

He shook his head, stopping me.

"That's something I have to live with. Something I will somehow have to deal with. But also losing my daughter...We haven't seen each other or talked to each other in more than five years. After med school, she came to Charlotte to finish a residency in Emergency Medicine. I thought...I thought that if I moved close by, I might have the chance to somehow connect with her. That's why Rock Hill seemed like such a good fit. I tried calling the ER at Charlotte Memorial over the last couple of months to see if she was working, hoping that she might pick up the phone even by mistake. But nothing. Seems like she avoids even a phone call. I've even thought about driving up and just walking in the ER one day. But that might create a scene, and I can't let that happen."

I remembered the recent phone call from the Charlotte Memorial ER. It had struck me then that it had been a little strange, and now I knew why. When I was handed the receiver, the secretary on the other end asked if this was Dr. Lesslie. I told her it was, and there was a hushed conversation in the background, and I heard 'Are you sure?' Then the secretary put the resident on the phone. Lexi MacLeod. Now I understood. She wanted to be sure it was me on the phone and didn't want to take the chance that it might be her father. I wasn't about to share this with Moss.

"That's why I'm here now, Robert. I've got to leave Rock Hill."

My heart sank. I had been trying to absorb all that he was telling me about his wife and daughter—trying to find the words I could use to somehow console him. Now, to learn that he was leaving, that was a blow I hadn't expected.

"I thought being in Rock Hill would be a good thing," he continued. "Don't misunderstand me. This is a great ER and a great staff. It's one of the best-run ERs I've ever seen, and it's been great working with you. It's just that...It's just that I can't be this close to my daughter and still be a world apart."

I saw the pain in his eyes and was beginning to understand. I tried to imagine what I would do in his situation, how I would act, where I would go. There was no answer. Moss had only been with us a brief six months, yet his leaving the ER would be a huge loss for everyone who worked with him. I wanted him to stay, but it wasn't up to me to offer him forgiveness or to bridge the chasm between him and Lexi. I was helpless.

"When are you thinking about making this change?" I asked him.

"I've only got two shifts left this month, and I've been able to get them both covered. After that...I know it's short notice, and I apologize, but Robert, I need to leave."

That was sudden. My mind flew to the gaps in the schedule and what that would mean for me and the rest of the staff. But I refocused on the man in front of me—I had to. His eyes were pleading, and he was hurting and needed relief. Any problems with the schedule were nothing compared to what he was dealing with.

"I understand, Moss. I'm sorry to hear this. Sorry to hear you're leaving and sorry to hear about your relationship with Lexi. I hope that will someday heal."

"I hope so too. But...I don't know."

He stood and stretched.

"We'll make it work here," I told him. "You do what you need to do."

"Thanks, Robert. I'll try to stop in before I leave town."

I watched as he walked out through Triage and out of the ER. I was numb, deflated, and wanted to go home.

Moss never came back by the ER. None of us saw him before he left town, and none of us learned where he might have gone.

Over the next six months, I spoke to Lexi MacLeod several times about patients we were sending her way. She never asked about her father, and I never mentioned his name.

> *To forgive is to set a prisoner free and discover that the prisoner was you.*
>
> —Lewis B. Smedes

7

A Seed Planted

Let me know if this hurts," I told the 58-year-old man sitting on one of our Ortho beds. He had slipped on some ice on the way to his car and landed on an outstretched hand. His right wrist was swollen and looked like it should be painful. I examined it gently.

"Not too bad, Doc. But it does hurt." He looked up and cocked his head. "You remember me?"

Maybe teachers and police officers have an easygoing response, but I can assure you that ER doctors tremble a little when asked this question. *How does he know me? Where did we meet? Did I make a mistake years ago? He's walking and talking, so that's a good thing.*

I studied his face, searching for some gleam of recognition.

He rescued me by saying, "Your wife had that Teens Under Fire program that I brought my 13-year-old to one time. I was the guy standing in the back of the room that almost passed out. Heck, I think I *did* pass out."

"Robert, there's been something on my heart, and we need to talk about it."

I braced myself. This could mean that my wife wanted me to

organize my sock drawer, throw away the half of my knit shirts that I never wore, or something worse.

I turned to her and said, "Sure, Barbara. What is it?"

Having four children, with the oldest two in middle school, Barbara knew the challenges of the teen years that lay in the all-too-soon future. She had been burdened with the idea of reaching out to troubled teenagers and offering them real choices, based on the experiences of others—many who had made the bad ones and learned painful lessons. It was a burden that she had tried to unload, tried to turn aside and bury. The Lord had other ideas.

"I woke up in the middle of the night, and it all came together. Crystal clear, and I know what I need to do."

She explained her vision of a program designed to help troubled teenagers—any teenagers. She even had an idea of what it should be called. Teens Under Fire—TUF.

"I don't want it be something like 'Scared Straight.' It needs to be tough, honest, and real. But I want to stress to as many kids as we can reach that they have importance and uniqueness and a place in this world. And I want to be able to share the gospel with them—to share Jesus."

It took several weeks to hammer out the particulars, but at each step of the way, doors opened, and TUF began to take on a life of its own. The county solicitor's office was supportive and planned to make the program part of the correctional requirements for juvenile offenders. That was a captive audience, and when the word got out, parents across the area wanted to have their children attend. She had to cap the number of teenagers in each session to 20—a number that was quickly filled.

TUF initially met once a month. The need was great, and this was soon increased to every two weeks. All told, the program lasted ten years and reached more than 2,000 teenagers. It was a lot of work for Barbara and the people who helped her.

It started on a school day, midafternoon, and lasted several hours. For most of that time, we started in one of the meeting rooms of Rock Hill General. The administration had graciously given us the opportunity and even allowed me to take the group through the ER, assuming it was quiet enough at the time. This was before HIPPA and would never be allowed today. Regrettably.

A typical gathering would include 18 to 20 teenagers and a few of their parents. We started with a slide program that I put together—pictures of crushed automobiles from a DUI, broken forearm bones from a baseball bat attack, elderly faces beaten to an unrecognizable pulp by teenage assailants. Graphic stuff. And it got their attention—or at least some of them. I noticed more than a few pairs of glazed-over eyes—usually among those who had been required to attend. But most of the kids were paying attention.

Then Barbara had a group of individuals who would take turns sharing their own life experiences. These were young and old adults who had experienced the ravages of alcohol and drugs—damaging not only themselves but those around them. Lost jobs, broken homes, severed relationships. This was real stuff and painful to hear. But more painful to tell. And there were those who had chosen a path of illegal activities of various descriptions and had been caught and punished. Again, destruction of families and drastically altered lives and opportunities.

"Don't make the mistakes I made."

Some of the kids listened and seemed to understand. Some just sat there. The sad reality is that only a few of us can learn from the mistakes of others. Most of us are stubborn, willful, and destined to find our way into the muck.

Next, she had arranged to have a group of incarcerated juvenile offenders—the insiders—who came up from Columbia. These were young men who openly shared the problems they had had and their experiences being locked up. Some would "graduate" from the juvenile facility to the "Big House," yet they wanted to make a difference. They wanted to share what they had learned with other teens who might be following right behind them. These were engaging and bright young men, and each had a story to tell. If they didn't think the kids were paying attention, they didn't hesitate to call them out. They'd get a few questions after their talk, and they didn't sugarcoat their answers. That night they'd be back behind bars, and they wanted the group to know what that felt like.

At that point, I would call around to the ER to see if the Trauma room was empty. Midafternoon, middle of the week—we usually had a good chance. I would lead the group as quickly and as quietly as possible to Trauma, shepherd them into the 20-by-20 space, and have them surround the stretcher, strategically located in the middle of the room. The door was closed, and I asked for a volunteer. Once or twice, a couple of hands would shoot into the air. Usually, there was only silence, and the kids just stared at each other.

If no one volunteered, I tried to pick out the most daring of the group and asked them to jump onto the stretcher and lie down.

"We're going through a scenario of something that we see all too often in this ER," I began. "We're going to pretend that...what's your name?...okay, Tyler has been out with some of his friends. It's a Saturday night. Someone bought a couple of six-packs, and they were over at the park. Some other guys came up, and there was an argument. Someone flashed a gun, and it went off, hitting Tyler right here."

I pointed to his mid abdomen, and he jumped. There was a chuckle from the back of the room, and I shot an icy glare in its direction.

"Nothing funny about this," I told them. "A bullet wound here can cause a lot of damage. Lots of stuff lying underneath it. Fortunately for Tyler though, his blood pressure was good and he was breathing. No other bullet wounds, which is something we always need to check for. He would have felt the first one, but maybe not the second...or the third. Even though he was stable, he would need to go to the OR and have his abdomen explored. Again, lots of things under that hole. The surgeon was called in, took a look at Tyler, and then called the OR. 'I'll let you know what I find, Robert,' he told me."

The room was quiet—no more chuckles from the back.

"I want to tell you something that happened—something I'll never forget. Two nurses came into Trauma and got Tyler ready to roll to the OR. They were almost to the doorway with him when he raised his hand. They stopped, and he looked up at me. 'Doc, I'm not going to make it.' I stopped writing on his chart, stunned, and looked down at him. I told him he was going to be fine, that he had a great surgeon, and I'd check on him later when he was out of recovery. 'I'm not going to make it,' he repeated."

Three hours later, the surgeon walked up the hallway and stopped beside me. He pulled off a sweaty cap and tossed it into a nearby trash can.

"That was tough," he told me. "That bullet nicked his aorta, and it had clotted off, but just as we opened him up, the clot came loose, and blood was everywhere. The hole was above his renal arteries and hard to get to. Finally got it cross-clamped, and we ended up giving him eight units of blood. But, Robert, we lost that boy. He had one cardiac arrest that we got him back from, but then he had another. Worked on him for more than an hour, but finally had to quit."

The two of us stood there in silence. After a moment, the surgeon sighed. "Does he have any family here?"

I let these words sink in, and after a moment of our own silence, I would walk to the door, turn to the group, and say, "Follow me. But no talking."

We quickly made our way down the back corridors of the hospital, past the service elevators, across the rear loading dock, and down a hallway lined with boxes of supplies. It was dusty and nowhere near as bright and clean as the rest of the hospital.

We stopped in front of a large wooden door, emblazoned in red letters with the word *MORGUE*.

When I had the attention of the group, I would ask them to describe this area of the hospital. Eyes flitted up and down the dank corridor. Occasionally, someone would say something like, "We're in the storage area," or "This place is spooky." Most often, there was only silence. I would point out to them the areas we had passed through—places in the hospital where no patients or visitors frequented. We had walked across a loading dock—just like the loading dock of any company or business. Things came in a truck and were unloaded. And things were loaded into vehicles and taken away. The difference here was that sometimes those *things* were the bodies of dead people.

"This is the morgue," I would tell them. "There might be some bodies in here, but don't worry. You won't see them."

Pushing open the door, I guided them into an area that contained two rooms. The first was a space surrounded on two walls with what appeared to be horizontally stacked refrigerators— three or four high. They were refrigerators. Once everyone was in the room and the door was closed, we passed into the area where autopsies were performed. It smelled of chemicals, and the bright lights cast an earthly glow upon the large metal stretcher standing starkly in the middle of the space. The top was constructed so that any liquids would drain to the center and down through piping into the floor. On the counters surrounding the room lay various instruments—large scissors, blades, strange cutting instruments, and scales.

"This is where autopsies are done. If we need to know a person's cause of death, one of the pathologists will examine the body, weigh all of the organs, take specimens for microscopic slides, and try to figure things out. Doesn't take long."

By this time, every eye in the room was on the table.

"Now let's go back into the other room."

The group shuffled slowly into the first space—the one with the refrigerators.

"This is where the bodies of dead people are stored, either waiting for an autopsy or for someone from a funeral home to pick them up."

We would always check beforehand to make certain which of the refrigerators were empty. I would walk over to one of these and open it for all to see. A metal rack easily slid out, allowing for the placement or removal of a body. There was frequently a soft gasp as it clicked into place.

"Let me tell you about this room." At this point, I would pick out one of the kids—usually a teenage girl—and tell this true story:

"A few weeks ago, there was a bad car accident out on Highway 21. Four teenagers were out late at night, and a guy, 19 years old had been driving. His girlfriend was in the passenger seat, unbelted. He lost control and went off the side of the road, running head-on into a tree. She was thrown through the windshield and across the hood of the car. Killed instantly. The driver has some scratches on his forehead and some sore muscles, but he walked away. The two in the backseat were belted and had only some minor injuries. EMS brought three of them to the ER to be checked out. They took one to this room and put her in that refrigerator."

I stopped here and pointed to one of the refrigerators directly behind them. Every eye turned in that direction. Silence.

"A little later, I had to walk her parents down that dark hallway into this room to identify their daughter. They knew what had happened, and you can imagine the pain they were in. Her mother said, *'She left the house about seven o'clock. Told us she loved us, and we told her to be careful. We never thought that would be the last time...'*"

I paused and stepped through the group to the front of the refrigerator. Grasping the handle, I pulled it open and slid out the tray.

"She was covered with a sheet, and I had to pull it off her head so her parents could see. She was a beautiful girl, with not a mark on her face. We stood here for a couple of minutes. They were devastated—their lives forever changed. And I had no words of comfort."

Silence in the room, and sometimes a few tears. The most anguished faces I saw were those of the parents in our midst. They knew what this would feel like.

I slid the tray in and closed the door.

"Then we left," I told the group. "Turned off the lights, closed the door, and left their daughter in a refrigerator. This should never happen. Never. But it does."

We led the group back to the meeting room, and Barbara finished the session telling them that they were special—each and every one of them. That God had a purpose for them, and that they had a place in His world. There were paths to choose—those that led to life, and those that led to misery, pain, and death. "Choose life," she told them.

I stood beside the Ortho stretcher, writing up the chart of our patient with the injured wrist. We'd get an X-ray, but I knew what we'd find, and I told him so.

"Yeah, that's what I expect," he said. "But this is good in a way. If I hadn't fallen and come to the ER, I wouldn't have had the chance to see you and to thank your wife. My son, Charlie, was getting into a lot of trouble back then. Running with the wrong crowd, getting hold of their parents' alcohol, and got busted for shoplifting. That's what got him sent to the Teens Under Fire thing. He *had* to go, and I went along to be sure he did. Anyway, while we were all in the Trauma room, and you were telling about that young guy with the gunshot wound...it got to me, and my head started spinning. The next thing I knew, I was sitting on the floor, and one of your nurses was fanning me. Boy, was Charlie embarrassed. I thought that was the only thing he remembered from that day.

"We continued to have trouble with him, and he barely made it out of high school. Tried York Tech for a year but gave that up. And for all those years, he still messed with alcohol and then with drugs. Didn't get arrested again, but came close. Things got so bad that the wife and I had to kick him out of the house. He has two younger sisters, and he was a bad influence. We tried to support him as best we could, but he would have to make a go of things on his own."

He paused and shook his head. "You just never know. Back when he was 13 at the hospital sitting through your wife's program, I was sure everything was passing into one ear and out the other. But when he was 22, he came by the house and wanted to talk. He wanted to talk about that Teens Under Fire program, and about how he should have paid attention to those people who were only trying to help him. He wished he had listened to how alcohol and drugs can ruin your life, because he learned it the hard way. In a bad way.

"He reminded me about my passing out in the back of the room, and we laughed. But then he told me what you had said about that young man with the gunshot wound, about how he was talking to you one minute and dead the next. It scared me when he told me, but he said he had come real close to being in that same situation—a couple of times.

"Whatever he remembered and whatever was in his heart, he was a different person. He was committed to changing the path he was on, and he did. He got a business degree from Winthrop and is working out at Catawba with Duke Power. He's married now, and has two kids of his own. Our first grandchildren. It's a great thing."

His voice trembled, and he cleared his throat. "Tell your wife he *was* listening. And tell her thank-you."

> *A farmer went out to sow his seed. As he was scattering*
> *the seed, some fell along the path, and the birds came*
> *and ate it up. Some fell on rocky places, where it did not*
> *have much soil. It sprang up quickly, because the soil*

was shallow. But when the sun came up, the plants were scorched, and they withered because they had no root. Other seed fell among thorns, which grew up and choked the plants. Still other seed fell on good soil, where it produced a crop—a hundred, sixty or thirty times what was sown. Whoever has ears, let them hear (Matthew 13:3-9).

Suck It Up

The ER—Wednesday, 5:30 p.m.

Lori Davidson wheeled an eight-year-old boy into the department. She had placed a splint and ice bag on his right wrist, and she looked over at me as they passed the nurses' station.

"Ortho," she said quietly. "Looks like a fracture."

She headed down the hallway to the Orthopedic room, followed by a man and woman who I assumed were the boy's parents. The man looked around the department and huffed loudly as he passed me. The woman walked a few steps behind. She kept her head down and cast furtive glances from side to side.

"Now that's strange," Amy Connors said when they were out of earshot. "A little peculiar, if you ask me."

I had noticed the same thing—the interaction, or lack thereof, between the two people we thought were the boy's mother and father.

Lori pushed the empty wheelchair to the nurses' station and slid the boy's chart onto the countertop.

"Looks like a buckle fracture," she told me. "His father says he fell on it while playing football, but it may have happened four or five days ago. Just now getting it looked at."

"Five days?" Amy echoed in surprise. "What took them so long to bring him in?"

Lori sighed and looked at me. "I think you'll understand when you talk to the father. And don't expect to get too much from the mother."

Lori was right about the boy's mother. She never said a word during the entire time they were in Ortho.

"Okay, Danny, tell me what's going on here."

I dropped the boy's chart onto the stretcher beside him and carefully picked up his still-splinted right forearm and wrist.

He didn't say anything. He was staring at his wrist and then looked up at his father.

"I'm Bill Truesdale, Danny's father. Danny was practicing football, and I'm one of the coaches of his team, I didn't actually see what happened. But he told me he was running and fell and landed on his right hand. He's complained of pain since, so we brought him in to be checked."

"Hmm. Well, let's take a look at this, Danny."

I slowly unwrapped the ACE bandage, removed the splint, and held Danny's small wrist and forearm. He grimaced a little with the movement.

"Sorry," I told him. "I'll hold it as still as I can. Just need to see where you're hurting."

"Tough it up, boy," his father said. "Let the doctor do what he needs to do."

I looked up at Bill Truesdale. A scowl spread across his face, and he folded his arms across his chest. Behind him, his wife took a step back, bumping into the supply cabinet.

"He's doing fine," I said, returning my attention to Danny's injured arm.

Lori was right. The back of his wrist was swollen and tender to the touch—just what you'd expect to find with a "buckle" or "greenstick" fracture. At his age, it would not be a through and through break, but would be a fracture, nonetheless, and would require treatment.

"Let's get a couple of X-rays and see what we've got."

"That's why we're here," Truesdale muttered.

I looked over at him, studying this impatient man.

"When did this happen?" I asked him.

He shuffled his feet and dropped his gaze to the floor.

"Like I said, he fell during football practice, and we're here to get it fixed."

I kept my eyes fixed on him, waiting for an answer to my question.

"It happened last Friday."

It was Danny, his voice quiet and quivering.

His father jerked around and put a hand on the boy's shoulder.

"It hasn't been that long," he said, staring down at his boy. "A couple of days, maybe. We just thought it was a bruise or something, and that it'd get better. Like I said, I'm one of the coaches, and I've seen a lot of injuries. Almost all of the time they turn out to be nothing—just a simple bruise or strain. No sense in making a big deal out of it. When I was growing up, my dad always told me to 'suck it up' and get on with things. Worked for me, and that's what we expect the kids on our team to do. Suck it up."

Danny's mother was silent.

I wanted to say something but caught myself. This wasn't child abuse, but it certainly bordered on neglect. The age of the bruising was consistent with five days, and that's a long time to sit on what should obviously be recognized as a probable fracture. Bill Truesdale was an intelligent man, but his macho attitude had caused his son unnecessary pain.

"We'll get some X-rays and get this taken care of."

Danny's films confirmed Lori's diagnosis and my own suspicion. He had a buckle fracture of his distal radius. He would need splinting, but no manipulation of the fracture. As long as he kept it still, it should heal without any problems. And at his age, an X-ray in a year or so would be completely normal—you'd be unable to see where the break had been.

"How long will he need to be in a cast?" his father asked.

"Well, as long as he keeps it in the splint we're going to put on him, he won't need a cast. Just something to keep that wrist from moving. That will help the pain as well."

"I'm not worried about the pain," he snorted. "He can handle that. If it's just a splint, he should be able to practice and play in Friday's game, right?"

I turned to the man and felt my face flush.

"Let's go over this again," I began slowly, measuring my words. "Danny has a fractured wrist. It's broken. And while this should heal without any problems, we have to...*you* have to take care of it. That means protecting it in a splint for three to four weeks. We're going to make that four weeks, and then he'll need to follow up with an orthopedist. But no contact sports until then. No football practice or games. Nothing."

Truesdale huffed and shook his head.

"He's our best linebacker. I guess we'll have to…Four weeks? That will be most of the season. Any way it could be less than that?"

Danny's mother was standing by the boy's side, gently stroking the back of his head. Silent.

"It's possible this greenstick fracture could become complete—break all the way through with additional stress. Then we'll have a whole different problem. So no, four weeks in the splint and no contact."

A huge sigh and then, "Well, do what you've got to do, doctor. We need to get out of here."

Danny whimpered once while we applied his form-fitting splint.

"Better?" I asked him, releasing his arm and watching as he held it before him.

He swung it around a little and said, "Yeah, that's better."

I turned to his mother. "Just be sure he keeps it on most of the time. He can take it off to bathe, but that's it. And no contact sports."

She nodded and reached out to help her son off the stretcher.

"Okay, let's go," his father said, glancing at his watch. "We've been here more than two hours. I've got to get to practice."

Lori met me in the doorway of Ortho with a wheelchair, and I scooted past.

"He won't be needing that," I heard his father tell her. "Come on, Danny. Let's go."

I reached the nurses' station and began writing on the boy's chart, documenting what we had just done for him.

"Well, look at that," Amy remarked.

I looked up at her and followed her glance to my left. The Truesdale family was walking up the hall with Lori behind, pushing the empty wheelchair.

"What do you mean?" I asked her.

"Look at the boy," she whispered.

During Danny's entire visit I hadn't seen him stand or walk. He was either in a wheelchair or on the exam table. He was walking up the hallway now, and I saw what Amy was referring to.

He was limping. It was a classic "antalgic" gait, with his "stance" phase—the part of your gait where your foot plants on the ground—being markedly shortened. He was getting off that foot as quickly as he could, indicating his avoidance of pain somewhere in that extremity. He was favoring his right leg, and something was going on.

I picked up his chart and stepped in front of the family.

"Danny, tell me, what's going on with your leg?" I asked. Glancing at his record, I wanted to be sure I hadn't missed an elevated temperature—something that might indicate an infection. It was 98.6.

"His what?" his father pounced. "There's nothing wrong with his leg."

He grabbed his son by the shoulder and tried to push past me.

"Just a minute," I stopped him. "Danny, is your leg bothering you?"

Without looking up, the young boy nodded.

"Lori," I said, looking around Truesdale to the nurse standing behind him. "Let's get Danny back in that wheelchair so I can take a look at that leg."

"It's nothing," Truesdale objected. "He just bruised his leg playing football a few weeks ago."

"It's been a few *months*."

It was Danny's mother—the first words I had heard her speak—and I stared at her.

"Whatever," Truesdale muttered, shaking his head. "It's nothing. Just a bruise. He just needs to get over it and stop being a baby."

Lori's face flushed. She pushed the wheelchair between Danny and his father and helped the boy sit down. Even this motion caused him to grimace, and he looked up at his mother.

"Yes, Dr. Lesslie," she said quietly. "Please take a look at him. I've been concerned with his limping, but..."

"Fine," Truesdale huffed. "You stay here with him and waste your time. I'm going over to the school for practice."

He spun around and stomped out of the ER.

Relieved, I squatted before the boy and said, "Okay, let's take a look at that leg."

Some eight-year-old children are unable or unwilling to give a good history of their problem—where things hurt and how badly they hurt. Danny knew where the trouble was and pointed directly to his right hip. He wasn't sure when it had started. There hadn't been a fall or anything, and it hadn't happened during football.

"No fever or chills? No recent viral-type infections?" I asked his mother.

"No, nothing like that."

I examined the boy's hip, and he cringed when I tried to passively rotate the joint. Any movement hurt him.

"Okay, that's all," I said, patting his thigh. Looking up, I said, "Momma, we're going to need some more X-rays."

There are several things that can cause hip pain in a young child, most of which are serious and need to be diagnosed and treated. Danny was the right age for a couple of these, and his story fit one that I suspected. *Legg-Calve-Perthes Disease* is caused by the loss of blood flow to the head of the femur, where it fits into the hip socket. We're not sure why this happens—something called *avascular necrosis*—but it can steadily worsen and cause permanent deformity and persistent pain in that joint. The diagnosis can usually be made with simple X-rays.

When Danny was wheeled back into the department from Radiology, the techs took him to the same stretcher in Ortho he had been on earlier. I walked into the room with his X-rays and put them on the view box.

"Mrs. Truesdale," I said to his mother. "Let's take a look at these."

She walked over and stood beside me, studying the black and white images on the backlighted box. I flipped off the overhead lights.

His hips and pelvis were displayed, and I pointed first to his left hip.

"This is what a normal hip his age looks like," I explained, tracing with a finger the contours of his hip joint and femoral head.

"And this is where Danny's problem is." I moved my hand and pointed to his right hip. It was obvious. The head of his right femur had collapsed in on itself, the bony structure was grossly irregular, and it was entirely different from his left hip—the normal one.

"Oh..." she sighed, glancing quickly at her son and then back to his X-ray. "What does this mean?"

I explained to her the diagnosis and what would need to be done. His hip had deteriorated badly and would never be normal again.

"I'm going to call one of the orthopedists, and he'll probably need to be put in the hospital for a while."

She nodded slowly, and her hand covered her mouth.

"Could this...if we had..." she fumbled.

"We don't know what causes this problem," I told her again. "So nothing you did caused it. It just happens. Had we found out sooner..." I had to be careful here. "Usually, the sooner we find out, the better, and the sooner we can start treatment, the better. But making the diagnosis is not always easy or obvious. Now we know, and we know what needs to happen."

I flipped off the view box light and picked up Danny's chart.

"I'll go call the orthopedist," I told her, turning to the doorway.

"He's not a bad person."

I stopped and turned to face her.

"He's not a bad man, Dr. Lesslie. My husband just...he expects a lot from Danny. And he expects him to be tough, not to complain about...things. His father was the same way. He coached high school football and expected Bill to be just like he was— tough and never complaining. 'Suck it up,' he always told him. It's just the way he was raised."

There was a lot I wanted to say, but this wasn't the time or place, or the right person.

"I hear you, Mrs. Truesdale. Let me call that surgeon."

> *Every father should remember one day his son will follow his example, not his advice.*
>
> —Charles Kettering

All That Glitters

ER, this is Silver Springs Rescue, do you read me?"

The squawking radio grabbed our attention, and Amy, our unit secretary, reached for the receiver.

"This is the ER, Silver Springs. Go ahead."

Crackling static and some undecipherable words.

Silence. Then, "ER, we're on the way in with a 42-year male. Multiple bee stings with anaphylactic shock."

That got my attention, and Lori Davidson's. She picked up a notepad and held her hand out to Amy.

"Hold on. You need to talk with our nurse." She handed the receiver to Lori and rolled back in her chair.

"This is the nurse, Silver Springs. Tell me about this patient."

"Like I said, multiple bee stings. At least 30, maybe 40. Got hit everywhere, and he's in a lot of pain."

I circled my index finger in the air, and Lori nodded. "What's his heart rate and blood pressure? And is he breathing?"

"He's breathin'. Can't you hear him screamin'?"

There was muffled moaning in the background, and it might have been screaming. If so, that would be good.

"And his heart rate is around 100. Last blood pressure was 150 over 100."

Lori looked up at me. That *wasn't* anaphylactic shock or any other kind of shock. The Silver Springs Rescue Squad consisted of a group of volunteers—good people and well intentioned, but not very well trained. Their headquarters was at the far end of the county, and they only got the emergency calls that our EMS system could not cover.

"We've got some O2 going and should be at your place in 20 minutes. We'll let you know if anything changes. Roger and over."

"Rog..." Lori squinted and closed her eyes, barely catching herself. "10-4 Silver Springs. We'll expect you in 20."

She hung up the receiver and took a deep breath.

"What do you think *that* is?" she asked.

"I know what it is!" Chad Niven was standing behind us, unnoticed when he came out of the Cardiac room. The newest addition to our staff, he had finished his emergency medicine residency a little over two months earlier. Bright and friendly, he had all the information he needed in his brain, but it would have to be coupled with some in-the-trenches experience. He would get that in the Rock Hill General ER.

"With that number of bee stings, he could be getting ready to crash in any minute. We saw a video in one of our conferences about how a honeybee stings and leaves its stinger in place. Really impressive. The venom sac keeps pumping through the stinger, even after it's detached from the bee. Can go on like that for a while, injecting more and more venom into the patient and making it difficult to get ahead of the allergic reaction. They all have to be found and removed. Let me handle this guy when he comes in, okay?"

Lori looked at Chad and then at me.

"Sure, Chad. He's all yours." I wasn't going anywhere.

"My uncle has honeybees," Amy piped up. "He has about a dozen hives and has only been stung once in more than 20 years. He says the honeybee is usually pretty gentle and doesn't go after you unless you're really messin' with the hive or put your hand on one. They die after they sting you, so I guess they want to be selective."

"This guy must have really provoked them to have been stung that many times," Chad observed. "This will be interesting. Lori, we'll need to strip him naked as soon as he gets here."

"That's her specialty," Amy quipped.

The ambulance entrance doors opened, and Silver Springs Rescue rolled into the department. One volunteer guided the head of the stretcher, while the other pushed from behind. Lying on the stretcher, his head propped up, was a middle-aged man in obvious distress. He was wearing a sweat-stained T-shirt and blue jeans. His bare feet were swollen and dotted with red welts, as were his face and arms.

The lead volunteer thrust a chart in the air as they hurried past the nurses' station.

"Where do you want him?" he shouted.

Lori was standing in the hallway and pointed into Major Trauma. The stretcher and its attendants disappeared into the room.

"I've got this," Chad spoke, dropping the chart in his hands to the countertop. "Amy, call the lab and let's get an EKG. Stat!"

He stalked into Major Trauma, stethoscope in hand. I followed at a respectable distance.

Johnny Watts moaned as he was moved to the stretcher in the middle of Major Trauma. He was surrounded by members of our team who were placing electrodes on his chest, nasal oxygen prongs in his nose, and rubbing his right forearm with alcohol in preparation for starting an IV.

"What's his pressure now?" Chad barked.

"162 over 98," one of the techs responded.

Chad was standing at the head of the stretcher, writing on a notepad. He paused and looked at the tech. "What was that again?

She repeated the same numbers and added, "Heart rate is 102."

He shook his head and made some notes.

Lori had quickly undressed Johnny down to his underwear, exposing more of the red welts on his chest, abdomen, and upper thighs. Too many to count, but well over the 30 or 40 Silver Springs had reported.

The two volunteers were standing against one of the walls, staring wide-eyed at the controlled chaos. Within a matter of minutes, an IV was running, the cardiac monitor was beep-beep-beeping with a rapid but regular rhythm, labs had been drawn, and an EKG was in Chad Niven's hands.

"We'll get out of your way, Dr. Lesslie," one of them spoke. "Let us know how he does."

"I will, and thanks, guys. Good work."

They pushed their stretcher into the hallway and disappeared.

Chad stood over our patient and pressed his stethoscope over the man's lungs.

"Take some deep breaths."

Johnny complied, and after a few breaths said, "Doc, I need something for pain."

Chad raised one hand in the air. He couldn't listen to the man's breath sounds and understand what he was saying at the same time. None of us can.

He stood up straight, tucked the stethoscope into his coat pocket and said, "Lungs are clear. No wheezing. Sounds fine. Now, what were you saying?"

Johnny repeated his request for something for pain.

Chad turned to Lori and said, "Thirty of Toradol IV. We don't want to sedate him with anything stronger. He could crash at any moment."

Johnny's eyes widened, and his frightened stare shifted from Niven to Lori and back to Niven.

Lori hadn't missed this and patted him gently on his shoulder. "Don't worry, Mr. Watts. You're going to be fine."

"Oh," Chad added. "Fifty of Benadryl and 125 of cortisone IV. We'll hold on the epinephrine for now."

Good idea.

Johnny got almost immediate relief with the pain medication and relaxed under the effects of the Benadryl. Chad leaned over him and studied the welts on his face and chest, prodding gently with an index finger.

"Strange," he muttered. "I thought we'd be able to see one of those venom sacs, but nothing in these." He rubbed one of the welts and then scraped it with the edge of his fingernail. "And I don't feel anything." Johnny winced. "Nope. Nothing here."

I had edged closer to the foot of the stretcher and looked closely at one of the wounds. It was dime-sized, raised, and an angry purplish red. In the center was a black dot—the apparent site of where a stinger had entered. But there was no stinger and no retained foreign body. It looked painful, and it was strange indeed.

"Mr. Watts, can you tell us how this happened?" I asked him.

He slowly opened his eyes and looked at me.

"Sure, Doc. My Aunt Sally called me this afternoon cause she knew I was startin' to keep some bees down on the place. A friend of mine gave me a couple of hives. Said he was tired of dealin' with 'em, and I said I'd be glad to have 'em. He told me what to do, and they seem to be doing fine. Anyways, Aunt Sally said she had a swarm of bees in one of her cedar trees and asked if I wanted them. I called my friend, and he told me what to do, how to slip up on 'em with a box, spray some sugar water on 'em, and shake 'em out of the tree and into a box. They're supposed to be real calm when they swarm like that, and you want to go slow and make sure you get the queen. Great way to get a free hive. So I did what he said, but drove off without the bee suit he gave me. I remembered he said I probably wouldn't need one, if I made sure to spray them and go real slow."

He paused and looked at the multitude of red welts covering his body.

"My mistake," he sighed.

"Blood pressure's still good," the tech reported.

Chad stood by the stretcher, stroking his chin—waiting for something to do.

"Let's sit tight," I volunteered. "He's stable right now, and let's see how he does."

I took a look at the welts again. These were not typical honeybee stings.

Glancing over to the corner of the room, I noticed Johnny Watts's clothes lying in a pile where Lori had tossed them. I walked over and kicked them a couple of times, making sure that nothing was going to fly out and attack me. Nothing did, and I picked up his shirt and shook it a couple of times. Something fell on the floor at my feet. It wasn't moving—and that was good. I leaned over and studied the critter. A large and long black body, with a couple of golden rings. This was no honeybee. It was a black hornet. Mean and easily aggravated. I picked it up and rolled it over in my hand, impressed with the wicked-looking stinger.

Fortunately, the treatment would be the same—watch for signs of a significant allergic reaction and treat whatever symptoms he was having. Unlike the honeybee, which leaves its stinger behind, the sting of a black hornet is one and done, but very painful. At least we wouldn't be worried about a prolonged injection of venom from hidden stingers.

In my mind's eye, I suddenly saw Johnny quietly slipping up on what he thought was going to be a manageable cluster of honeybees. Setting his box on the ground beneath the cluster—actually, a grayish hive, covered with hornets—he would have sprayed the swarm with sugar water and then shaken the branch holding it. There's not a human on this earth that can outrun an angry swarm of hornets, and Johnny certainly wasn't able to. He was lucky to have escaped with the number of stings he had suffered.

I walked over to the stretcher and stood beside Chad. Without saying a word, I opened my hand in front of him.

"Is that what a honeybee looks like?" he asked, leaning his face within inches of my palm.

Johnny leaned forward and twisted his body so he could see.

"What? That ain't no honeybee!" he exclaimed. "That's a darned hornet! Wait 'til I get hold of Aunt Sally."

"A hornet?" Chad muttered. He reached into a coat pocket, pulled out a treatment manual, and started thumbing through its pages.

"You're going to be fine, Johnny," I told him. "Doesn't look like you're going to have any serious allergic reaction, but you're going to have some pain for a while. We'll help with that. And take it easy with your aunt. She made an understandable mistake. Lots of folks have done the same thing."

As Lori and I walked out of the room, she leaned close and whispered, "Did learning take place?"

Hmm...on a couple of levels. I hoped.

> *We all make assumptions every day. Some more important than others. Some more damaging than others. And things, very often, are not what they seem.*
>
> —B.B. Shepherd

Lean Not on
Your Own Understanding

The Charleston County ER was nothing like what I expected. I had been warned by some of my fellow med students that it was wild, crazy, and sometimes dangerous. The citizens from a four-county area filled its ER bays with gunshot wounds, stabbings, assaults with various and imaginative weapons, and overdoses of things I didn't know existed. I was expecting the worst, but this was worse than the worst.

As a second-year medical student, I was assigned to spend several weekend shifts in that ER, usually 12 hours in length, with some of them overnight. I was also told to see and learn what I could, but to stay out of the way. That was fine with me. I could name the small bones in the wrist and trace the circulation of blood from one side of the heart to the other, but if asked to treat a gunshot wound of the abdomen, I would be as useless as the *g* in *lasagna*.

On my second shift at the "County," I was safely distanced and watched as surgical interns and residents sutured an assortment of lacerations, cleaned and dressed facial lye burns inflicted by an angry ex-girlfriend, and observed with amazement the placement of a chest tube in a young man with four stab wounds into his left lung. All that in the space of about two hours.

At midnight, something happened that I'll never forget. The ambulance doors opened and in staggered a twentysomething-year-old male, barefooted and bare chested, wearing only tattered and soiled blue jeans. He stopped in front of the Triage desk and stared wildly around the department. For a split second, no one said a word. The man's face was covered in blood, and blood was dripping down his torso. What caused the momentary pause in the department was the hatchet impaled in the top of his head.

The place exploded into action. He was scooped up and carried into the Major Trauma room and deposited on a stretcher. A multitude of orders were loudly barked by several of the physicians, and nurses were frantically gathering anticipated supplies.

When he was stabilized as much as possible, the senior surgical resident called out, "Who's on for neurosurgery?"

The answer came back from the nurses' station. "Satterfield!"

"Satterfield?" the resident questioned. "What did we do to deserve him?"

I didn't know any of the medical staff and glanced at one of the junior residents, my eyebrows raised.

He nodded and said, "That's a good thing."

I didn't know it at the time, but it *was* a good thing. Brent Satterfield was a 45-year-old neurosurgeon, trained in some of the best centers in the country, and heavily courted to come to Charleston. He was in a practice with four other neurosurgeons—the premier group in the area, maybe in the entire Southeast.

"You'll see," the junior resident quietly added.

Twenty minutes later, Satterfield walked into Major Trauma wearing surgical scrubs and rumpled lab coat. His long, sandy hair, rugged features, and piercing blue eyes cast an imposing, self-assured presence.

"So, what do we have here?" he asked, walking over to the side of the stretcher.

"Are you the surgeon?" the young man asked. The small hand ax still protruded from the top of his head, anchored in the coronal bone of his skull. No one dared try to remove it.

"'Fraid so, son." He took the man's face in his large hands and studied the location and depth of the ax's blade. "Looks like you have a bit of a problem."

The man reached up, his hand nearing the handle of the hatchet. Satterfield gently but firmly grabbed his arm.

"We need to let that be for the time being. I'll need to look at your X-rays and see what we're dealing with. Then we'll be taking you to the OR. Do you have any family members here with you?"

The patient huffed and shook his head. "The only family I have is a brother, and he's the one who did this."

"Hmm," Satterfield mused. "Let's hope he's not here, right? Anyway, you're talking and everything is working. That's all good news. We just need to remove this ax, and you'll be fine."

"You think so, Doc? Really?"

"You'll be fine."

A little before 1:00 a.m., he was wheeled out of the department and to the OR. As if a switch had been flipped, the ER quieted down, and within an hour, every bed was empty. Earlier, I had the chance to see my first beet-red eardrum—the infected middle ear of a two-year-old with fever and an earache—and I was happy for that. But I was also happy that things had slowed down enough for the staff to take a break. The third-shift crew had come in—much reduced in number from the day and evening crews. The senior surgical resident was still there, but that was it. And me. No help at all.

We sat quietly behind the nurses' station and chatted a little about the patients seen over the past few hours. I didn't know enough to ask any pertinent questions, and after an hour passed with no new patients, the resident turned to the nurse on duty.

"I'm going to close my eyes in room 3. Holler if something comes in."

"Sure thing," she answered, getting up and walking to the medicine room to catch up on her charting.

That left me alone, wondering what might walk or be carried through those ambulance doors, and wondering what in the world I was doing here.

I had grown up in two small towns. First in Mount Holly, NC, until the age of 14. We then moved to Due West, SC (yes, that's a real place), where my father taught organic chemistry in a small liberal arts school—Erskine College. My education there had prepared me for the rigors of medical school, and I was enjoying the academic challenges that constantly presented themselves. Gross anatomy, physiology, pathology—all tangible subjects, requiring time and effort to manage, but they were manageable. What was alluding me was something intangible, something that I was seeking and hadn't yet found. In the midst of this "basic science," surrounded by a leading medical center and being instructed by physicians with national—sometimes international—reputations, I was searching for evidence of a connection between the hard facts we were learning and the spiritual side of our existence. Where did the study and practice of medicine connect with a person's faith? Our lectures were crammed with information—facts to memorize and file away. They would be needed for upcoming examinations and one day in our care of actual people. There seemed to be no time for considering the question of "Why?" or taking a moment to marvel at the intricacies of the human body and wondering how all of this came to be. There was too much to learn. Yet, I wanted to find someone who had considered all of this, and who might share his faith with his students. Someone who had connected the science of medicine with something much larger.

My father had done that. He was the son of a minister and after serving in Europe during the Second World War had earned his PhD in organic chemistry at MIT He had no problem seeing the hand of God in everything around him, whether it was in his garden or in his classroom. The seasons of the year were ordered, offering a time to sow and a time to reap, and the predictable outcomes of chemical reactions and the molecular structure of proteins had God's fingerprints all over them. In his mind, there was no dichotomy separating hard, visible science with the reality of the presence of the Creator in His creation. I also believed that, and I guess I was looking for some confirmation that there were esteemed, learned men and women in the medical sciences that believed it as well. I'm sure there were those around me who felt that way, but the evidence of that belief was not obvious, at least not to me. We were about the business of becoming physicians—endlessly assembling cold, hard facts, and determinedly blinded to anything that would interfere with that.

As I sat in the County ER, I reflected on the things I had seen during this shift. There was plenty of sickness and disease, and more than enough of the evidence of man's ability to seek to harm his fellow man. I had a glimpse of how all of this could cause a person to wall himself off from the surrounding misery and pain and just focus on what was in front of him. Treat the pneumonia. Sew up the lacerated face. Set and splint a fractured wrist. Maybe that was the answer. Become proficient in doing these things and stay focused only on that. Learn everything you can and someday be able to stand in an ER like this and handle anything and everything that finds its way through those doors. There would be time later to sort out what it all meant. Maybe.

Brent Satterfield walked up to the nurses' station, glanced around the department, and slumped into the chair beside me. He still wore a sweat-soaked surgical cap, and his shoe covers were splattered with blood.

He glanced at the embroidered stitching on the front of my lab coat. "Well...Robert, were you here when the buried hatchet came in?"

I told him I was and asked how things went in the OR.

"He's one lucky young man," he began. "The hatchet fractured part of his skull and penetrated into the dura, but there was no significant tissue damage. We had to clean up a good bit of dirt and debris, but he's awake and oriented. Unless things get infected, he's going to be fine. Live to fight another day."

"Have you ever seen anything like that?" I asked. Obviously, I hadn't and wondered how common an occurrence this might be.

"A hatchet?" he chuckled. "Nope. That's a first for me. Seen a lot of other stuff—bullets, knives, crowbars, not a few hammers, but never a hatchet. You just never know what people will do to each other."

He rolled his shoulders and tilted his head back, taking a deep breath.

"Long day," he sighed after a few moments.

He looked down at my name again. "So, Robert Lesslie—second-year medical student, I would assume. What's been the most difficult part of medical school for you thus far?"

I hadn't expected this question and had to collect my thoughts before answering. I was sleep deprived, maybe a little careless, and as soon as the words were out of my mouth, I realized my answer was not what he was looking for.

"I'm having a hard time putting all of this together."

"You mean connecting gross anatomy with a hatchet wound to the skull?" he chuckled again. "What layers of bone and tissue would be involved with this type of injury?"

"No, not that. I'm struggling with how this all fits together, what it all means, and how does what I'm seeing in this ER...what we do to each other...how is there room for God in all of this."

What a mistake. Here was an eminent neurosurgeon asking me a question about my medical school experience, and I...he's going to get up and walk out of here.

Satterfield sat upright in his chair and turned in my direction. For a long moment, he studied me, his eyes never leaving mine.

He nodded his head, took off his glasses, and laid them on the desk in front of us.

"Now, that's a good question. It's something I wrestled with for a lot of years, and I expect you might as well. But you're asking the right question, and I'll share what I've learned."

He settled back in his chair and stretched out his legs.

"When I started medical school, I had no idea what I wanted to end up doing. In fact, I really had no idea of the options before me. But throughout those years, I began to understand that surgery was something that really appealed to me—something I felt comfortable and challenged with. And then I spent some time with a neurosurgeon, and things just clicked. It wasn't that I chose neurosurgery. I think neurosurgery chose me. And it's been the best thing I could ever have done. There are a lot of troubling cases, to be sure. Things that I have no control over and people that I can't help. But when I can, when surgery can save a life or forestall a disaster, it's...well, that's what makes it all worthwhile. Yet, just like you, I wrestled with how to make sense of it all. How could I find Jesus in the operating room? It's Jesus we're talking about, right? Not some vague notion of a benevolent, impersonal, all-knowing spirit."

I nodded, and he continued.

"Usually, those thoughts came to me just as they are to you now—in the middle of the night in some ER or surgical lounge. And I bet, just like you, I looked for someone to lean on, someone to share this with."

I nodded, amazed that this stranger, this surgeon, was sharing these thoughts with me.

"Are you familiar with Martin Luther?"

The question surprised me, and I fumbled a response. "Yes. I know that he nailed a piece of paper on a church door in Germany and that he wrote 'A Mighty Fortress.'"

"Well, that's a start. It'll serve you well to study Luther's works. It has me. He has a lot to say about our 'reason,' about how our greatest stumbling block to understanding the nature of this world and the character of God is relying on our own wisdom, our own knowledge, and our own understanding. Don't get me wrong, Robert. We're given brains, and we're supposed to use them. But until we come up against something that stares us in the face and shows us how little we really know, we'll always be wearing blinders."

I shook my head. He sounded like my father.

"What?" he asked. "Doesn't ring true?"

"Yes, but I'm trying to put reason and faith together—here in this ER, and with that guy with the hatchet in his head."

"Okay, what if I put it this way? I *use* my reason, but I'm not *governed* by it."

He paused, and I thought about these words. *Not governed by it.* A light flickered, and my brain struggled to grasp this truth. Or maybe it was my heart.

"Let me tell you a story," he resumed. "And then I'll need to get out of here. Early on in my practice, just a few years out of residency, I had a difficult case with a 60-year-old man. He had a brain tumor, and I wasn't sure if it would be amenable to surgery. He and his wife were great folks, and I explained to them that I really wouldn't know until I was able to take a look. They were both very calm—somehow at peace with the whole thing. They understood the seriousness of what we were dealing with and that he might not survive surgery. And if he did, there might be nothing we could do. His wife proceeded to tell me about her own experience. She gave me my first real lesson in the fallibility of reason and logic."

Satterfield leaned forward and put his hands on his thighs.

"A few years earlier, she had found a lump in her breast and gone to see her family doctor. One thing led to another, and a breast biopsy was scheduled. The day before this was to happen, one of her close friends told her about her own experience with a breast mass. Her doctor had ordered a couple of mammograms and ultrasounds and was sure they were dealing with cancer. The morning of the biopsy, the surgeon prepped the area and was using an ultrasound to guide the needle aspiration. He took a long time doing this, and finally told the woman that he couldn't find the nodule. It wasn't there. Gone. Three days earlier it was easily seen—about an inch in diameter. But now it was gone. She attributed it to prayer and God's intervention. Then my patient's wife told me that when she presented for her own biopsy, and after long sessions of prayer, her fear and anxiety had quietly yielded to a sense of peace. That was an answer in itself. But when her surgeon prepared to do the needle biopsy, he also lingered, studying the ultrasound images, searching for the cancerous lump. It was gone. Just like her friend's. And she's had no problem since. Now, how do we make sense of that? How does our logic explain the disappearance of these lesions? It can't. We can try, but we can't. That's what I mean when I say that I use my reason, but I'm not governed by it."

He stopped and studied my face.

"What about your patient?" I asked, wondering if there was another miraculous healing here. "What about the man's brain tumor?"

"When we got to the OR, and I exposed the area of his brain containing the tumor, it was sitting right there in front of me. Malevolent appearing, and threatening to destroy this man's brain and life. But it had not yet spread its fingers into his cortex, and I was able to completely remove the tumor. Every bit of it. After more than 15 years, he's still cancer free. That too was an answer to prayer. My years of training had prepared me technically for that moment, but I had no idea of what I would find, and I had feared and expected the worst. Yet..."

He looked over in the direction of the ER entrance.

"Looks like you're about to get busy," he said, standing and putting on his glasses.

A young mother with three small children was being led by our Triage nurse into the department.

"Remember, Robert, finely hone your reason, but don't let it govern you."

He walked past the young family and into the night.

Over the next couple of years in Charleston, I would pass Brent Satterfield a few times in the hallways of the hospital or see him from a distance in the staff cafeteria. Once, when our eyes met, he nodded at me. We never talked again, but his words of that night in the County ER have remained with me. I hope that in the following years I have managed to hone my reason. And I struggle, usually with some small success, to not let it govern me.

> *Trust in the LORD with all your heart, and lean not on your own understanding; in all your ways submit to him, and he will make your paths straight* (Proverbs 3:5-6).

Holy Quietude

The Puritans used this phrase—*holy quietude*—to describe how Christ-centered inner peace should control our hearts and minds. If it had another name, it would be Sadie Thompson.

"What do you recommend, Sadie?"

I was standing in front of the hot-food counter in the hospital's dining room, trying to decide what I wanted to eat for lunch. Sadie Thompson stood on the other side, armed with a ladling spoon in one hand and a set of tongs in the other. Her faded and frayed apron was stained with three decades of cooking thousands of meals in the kitchen of Rock Hill General.

There was a gleam in her eyes, and a warm and radiant smile spread across her face. With the back of one hand, she tried without success to adjust the hairnet that had slipped down over her forehead.

"These darned things. I wish somebody would make one that'd stay on your head."

"Well, Sadie, you just move too fast," I kidded her. "I'm surprised it stays on at all."

Sadie and I first met in the ER when she brought her sister, Anna, in with fever and shortness of breath. Anna had pneumonia, but it was the metastatic breast cancer that was driving things and that would soon end her life.

Anna was lying on the stretcher in room 4, and Sadie was in a chair by her side. They both knew where things stood, and that treating the pneumonia would help, but only for a little while—a few weeks at the most. In spite of that, they both looked up at me with smiles on their faces as I walked into the room.

"Anna, it's what we thought. Your X-ray shows a pretty bad pneumonia. You'll need to come into the hospital for IV antibiotics so we can get ahead of this."

Anna nodded and looked up at her sister, then closed her eyes and whispered something. I made out the name Jesus, but that was all.

"Excuse me?" I asked, immediately realizing I had overstepped into a place that was not mine.

They both looked at me, and Anna said, "Turn your eyes upon Jesus."

"That's right," Sadie echoed. "We're going to be okay."

When I worked days in the ER and had time to get something to eat, Sadie seemed to always be there in the dining room. And I was always glad to see her. Three weeks after the ER visit with her sister, I was once again standing at the hot-food counter.

"Dr. Lesslie."

I was deep in thought, concerned with a couple of patients in the ER, and I was standing there looking off into space.

"You with us?" she prodded, smiling.

"Oh hey, Sadie," I responded. "Just trying to get some lunch."

"I want to thank you for your help with my sister, Anna. You remember when we were in the ER with pneumonia."

I did remember and told her so.

"Well, she got better with the pneumonia and made it home. But she passed not long after, about a week ago."

"I'm sorry to hear that, Sadie. It looked like the two of you were very close."

"We were, we were." She was still smiling and nodding her head. "She always had her eyes fixed on the Lord. Always turned her eyes upon Jesus. She's home now."

I was to hear that phrase from her many times over the following years—*Turn your eyes upon Jesus*—almost always shared over the counter in the dining hall, and always when I needed to hear it. Somehow, she knew when I was troubled or distracted, and she never failed to reach out.

It wasn't just to me that she reached out. She touched a lot of people in the hospital. And I'm sure she did the same in whatever circles she traveled.

But not everyone was interested in her words of comfort and assurance.

"This looks like crap!"

Sam Chisolm, one of the surgeons on staff, was standing in front of me at the hot-food counter. He stared down at the food and shook his head. "It always looks like crap."

I was looking at the same choices, and they didn't look too bad.

"Dr. Sam," she said, her voice calm, soothing. "The meatloaf is pretty good today. And the okra."

Chisolm leaned closer and stared at the food.

"Crap!"

He picked up his tray and stomped away.

Sadie looked after him and shook her head. "Hmm, hmm, hmm. Must have had a bad morning in the OR. He just needs a little grace."

He needed more than that, and I was about to say so when she looked at me and said, "Now, Dr. Lesslie, don't even say anything. I know just what you need."

I watched as she served a plate with exactly the things I was going to ask for. Strange how she knew that, and how she sensed my mood.

"And remember, turn your eyes upon Jesus."

I looked into her smiling eyes, and my spirit lifted. She couldn't know the nature of the problem I was dealing with, but she sensed that I was troubled by something. And she was right. I was in the midst of dealing with a thorny issue involving our CEO, one of my partners, and a physician in an outlying hospital. She knew.

"Thanks, Sadie. You nailed it right on the head."

It seemed like she worked every day in that kitchen. Or that's what it seemed like to me—always there for more than 15 years. Until she wasn't.

"Sadie's not working today?" I asked Rachel Gaston, the director of food services. It was noon, and she stood behind the hot-food counter, where Sadie reigned.

She tilted her head, and her shoulders drooped.

"You haven't heard, Dr. Lesslie?"

"Heard what?" I asked. A coldness crept over me, and I dreaded the answer.

"Sadie passed last week."

What? She was standing right here only a few weeks ago. I had worked a string of nights and hadn't been here for lunch.

"Yes, the cancer finally caught up with her. She worked as long as she could. Only stopped when she couldn't make it from the parking lot to the kitchen. She worked right up 'til three days before she died."

"Cancer," I stuttered. "I didn't know."

"She didn't want you to know," Rachel sighed. "Didn't want anyone to know. That's how she was. Always worried about other people and never about herself. Always at peace, and always shared that peace with anyone who would accept it. I'm going to miss her. We're all going to miss her. I know you will too. You were special to her."

"Special?" I stumbled. "I'm not sure how..."

"Just accept it and be glad. You were special to her."

I ordered something for lunch and walked away. There was a huge hole in my heart and an awful ache.

A few years after Sadie left us, I came across an ancient songbook and thumbed through its yellowed pages. I stopped when one of the titles caught my attention, and I read the verses and refrain of an old hymn. Sadie's hymn. She was once again standing before me, smiling, wearing her apron and waving a serving spoon. The words pierced my heart:

> *Turn your eyes upon Jesus, Look full in His wonderful face. And the things of earth will grow strangely dim, In the light of His glory and grace.*
>
> —Helen Howarth Lemmel (1863–1961)

Doing the Right Thing

The ER—Tuesday, 8:00 a.m.

"Robert, we need to talk."

Stanley Baker, the CEO of Rock Hill General Hospital, was standing beside me in the hallway of the ER. I was writing on a chart and hadn't seen him walk up.

"Sure, Stanley. Let me finish this and give it to the secretary."

I dropped the chart into the "Orders" basket, and he followed me up the hall into empty room 5.

"What's on your mind?" I asked him.

He pulled the curtain closed, folded his arms across his chest, and leaned against the stretcher.

"One of your doctors, Brad Hayes, has been causing some problems."

Problems? Brad was one of the best doctors we had, and I struggled to imagine how he could be causing problems for this administrator.

"What do you mean?" Without thinking, I folded my own arms across my chest and stood a little straighter.

"It seems he has a problem with one of the surgeons at Divine Mission Hospital. He got in touch with their chief of staff and complained about him. That physician went straight to Jasper Jenkins, the administrator there, and reported what was going on. Jasper called me at home last night and gave me an earful. He wanted to know why my ER doctors were meddling in the affairs of his hospital and demanded that it stop immediately. I didn't know what to say. I told him I didn't know anything about it, but that I'd check into it and make sure it stopped. I know you're aware that we get a lot of patients from that hospital, and we need to stay on good terms with them. I don't know what's gotten into Dr. Hayes, but you'll need to rein him in. Immediately."

This didn't sound like Brad. If he had taken this kind of action, he must have had a good reason. There would be an explanation, and I needed to find it.

"Let me talk with Brad and see what's going on. He's coming in this afternoon, and I'll let you know what I find out."

"Just be sure this gets resolved by the end of the day," Baker replied. "I don't need this kind of heartburn."

He pulled the curtain aside and left the ER.

Divine Mission Hospital is a small facility—less than 50 beds—located 25 miles from Rock Hill. We get a lot of calls for advice from their ER doctors. A lot of their patients are beyond the capability of their ER or hospital to handle, and they send them our way. The hospital didn't have a large medical staff. It had only one general surgeon, Francis Looper, and only a few weeks ago, I had seen one of his patients in our ER.

"Mr. Jacobs, I'm Dr. Lesslie. What can we do for you this morning?"

It was a Saturday, and 46-year-old Billy Jacobs was lying on the stretcher of room 4. The chief complaint noted on his chart was "hernia."

"I guess I need a second opinion, Doc."

He was in a hospital gown and pulled it up to reveal his abdomen—crisscrossed with what appeared to be surgical scars.

"I had a hernia a couple of years ago—happened at work when I was lifting a heavy crate. Inguinal, I think they called it." He pointed to one of his scars and said, "This was where they operated on it. About a year later, it came back." He traced another of the incisions and continued, "And this was the next operation." Billy sat up and studied his belly. "This one was the last operation, when the hernia came back again. About three months ago."

As he sat up, I had noticed a bulge in the middle of this scar. An incisional hernia, protruding because of the increased intra-abdominal pressure caused by his sitting up. *What a mess.*

I examined his abdomen and the latest incision. There was a significant defect in the muscle wall—another hernia that would need to be repaired.

"You mentioned a second opinion," I said. "What do you mean?"

"Well, I saw my surgeon last week, and he told me I needed another operation. My wife wants me to get another opinion, and I just came over here."

None of the surgeons in Rock Hill would have done any of this, and I asked, "Where did you have this done? And who's your surgeon?"

"It's Dr. Looper over at Divine Mission," he answered, pulling his gown over his abdomen. "I know it's not an emergency or anything like that. I just needed some help with figuring out what to do."

I pulled up a stool and sat down. "Don't worry about that, Mr. Jacobs. That's why we're here. Let me just ask this: If Dr. Looper had operated on you three times for the same thing and it still isn't right, do you really want him operating on you again?"

Billy sighed and shook his head. "You sound just like my wife."

We made a referral to one of the surgeons in town.

"Brad, tell me what's going on with this Dr. Looper over at Divine Mission Hospital."

Brad Hayes had just walked up to the nurses' station and grabbed the chart of the next patient to be seen. His faced flushed, and he dropped the chart to the countertop.

"Robert, I haven't had a chance to talk with you yet, but I had a case the other night that was the final straw. It was a guy who came in after being seen in the ER at Divine Mission—seen by the surgeon on call and sent home. It was a disaster, and not the first one from down there. I mentioned it to Chuck, and he's had the same experience. A couple of them. I didn't know what to do, but felt like I had to do something. The surgeon there is a guy named Francis Looper, and he's dangerous."

Chuck Miller was another of our ER doctors—well trained, levelheaded, and not given to hyperbole or emotional outbursts.

"We see strange stuff all the time," Brad continued. "And we just handle it. But something's going on in that hospital, and things have piled up over the last few weeks—all involving this Looper guy—and I just had to do something."

"Tell me about it."

One thing an ER doctor quickly learns (or he/she *better* learn) is that we all live in glass houses. Everything we do is visible to other doctors, to the nursing staff, and to the administration. Not so much for other physicians—family practitioners, internists, pediatricians—whose mistakes, if they make them, occur in the relative privacy of their offices. Surgeons live in glass houses as well, with most of their critical work done in the operating room. That's why you talk with the OR staff if you want to know who's the best technical surgeon/orthopedist on staff. And if you live in a glass house, you've got to be careful when you throw stones. It can come back to bite you.

Brad Hayes was throwing stones. He knew the reality of our glass house, but he was hurling them just the same. As it turned out, he had good reason.

He proceeded to tell me about several patients he had seen recently in the ER, all having been treated by Francis Looper at Divine Mission.

"When I mentioned Looper to Chuck, he just shook his head and told me about two people he had seen in the past two weeks—both mishandled by that guy."

"Let me tell you about the first patient of his I saw," Brad began. "Probably three weeks ago, in the middle of the night."

Brad shared his experiences with me. All of us are human, and we all make mistakes. But when he finished, I was stunned.

The first patient was a 60-year-old man who came to our ER with abdominal pain. His history was classic for appendicitis—right-lower-quadrant pain, nausea, some vomiting, and a low-grade fever. He mentioned that he had been seen by a surgeon in the ER of Divine Mission the day before. The surgeon told him that his white count was elevated, but there was nothing bad going on. He was sent home and got worse.

When Brad examined his abdomen, he found exquisite right-lower-quadrant pain and rebound (an indication of inflammation/irritation within the abdomen). It was a straightforward diagnosis, and as Brad was about to pull the sheet back over the man, he noticed a strange puncture wound overlying his right upper abdomen. He gently palpated the area and studied the small clot. There was another on the left side. And two more over the lower abdomen—one on the right and one on the left.

"What happened here?" he asked.

"Oh, that's where the surgeon stuck me with a needle and syringe. Told me he was looking for pus, and when he didn't find any, he said I was fine. Hurt like the dickens."

A four-quadrant tap! It was something I had come across in an ancient surgical manual—something from the medical Dark Ages. Nobody did this anymore—not in decades. Totally useless and potentially dangerous. He did, in fact, have a hot appendix—at the point of bursting. He was operated on in our hospital and went home without any problems.

The next patient didn't fare as well. He had been seen in the ER of Divine Mission after having suffered a 220-volt electrocution while working at a local manufacturing plant. The ER doctor noted an apparent entrance wound over his right palm and an exit wound near the right shoulder and then had asked Dr. Looper to evaluate this injury. Looper spent less than two minutes with him, asked the ER doctor why he had been called for such a trivial matter, and wrapped the man's arm with an ACE bandage.

"You'll be fine," he told him. "Take some Tylenol if you have any pain, and give it a couple of days."

The man was *already* in significant pain, but he went home, only for things to get worse. Two days later, he showed up in our ER with a tense and swollen right forearm.

"It was the worst compartment syndrome I've ever seen," Brad said. "His hand was white as a piece of paper and cold. No pulses. He was crying in pain."

Electrical injuries can be subtle—no initial symptoms early on, but if the current passes through muscles and other underlying structures, significant damage can be done. Swelling follows, with compression of nerves and loss of blood flow. If not recognized and treated, muscles die and irreparable damage occurs. It's called a *compartment syndrome*. Brad recognized what was going on, but it was too late. In spite of aggressive treatment, the man lost most of the muscles in his forearm and use of his right hand. It didn't need to happen. Tylenol and "Call me in the morning" wouldn't get it.

The next person Brad told me about had a similar story, also involving electricity. This one had to do with a lightning strike.

Pete Jenkins was playing golf with his usual foursome, when out of nowhere a thunderstorm materialized. The sky darkened, the wind picked up, and thunder began booming all around them. Pete was out in the middle of the fairway when a bolt of lightning blazed across the sky and knocked him to the ground.

"I thought I was dead," he later told Brad. "There was a terrible smell, and I remember reading that some people describe an ozone smell, whatever that is. But this was more like burning flesh."

Pete had gone to the closest ER—Divine Mission—and was evaluated by the ER doctor on duty. Pete's right golf shoe was blackened, and his right foot was causing him a lot of pain. While one of the nurses began cutting away the shoe, the ER doctor ordered an EKG and asked their secretary to call in Dr. Looper.

Looper happened to be in the hospital and walked into the ER a few minutes later. One of the techs was placing electrodes on Pete's chest, arms, and legs, and was about to turn on the machine to run an EKG.

"Hold on there," Looper stopped her. "What are you doing that for?"

The ER doctor looked at Looper and said, "I ordered an EKG to make sure the electrical activity of his heart is stable. There's no question he was struck by lightning, and that's one of the..."

"Forget that," Looper interrupted. He walked over to the stretcher and started ripping the electrodes off of Pete's chest. "We won't be needing this. He's breathing, isn't he? I'll take over now."

The ER doctor gave up and left the room.

"That doctor ripped my sock off and almost killed me!" Pete Jenkins later explained in our ER. "He poked my foot a couple of times, said I'd be fine, and told me to go home and put some ice on it. That's about the time my wife got there, and we got straight in the car and drove to Rock Hill."

"It's a good thing his wife did that," Brad told me. "I looked for an entrance and exit wound, but only saw damage to his right foot. By the time he got here, his foot was pale, and I couldn't find a pulse. There was a wound about the size of a quarter, and this strange, feathery-type rash around it."

"A lightning print, some people call it," I observed.

"Yeah, I've read about that, and that's exactly what it looked like. We *did* get an EKG, and it was fine. And while he was in the ER, he started complaining of a ringing in his ears. I did a quick assessment of his hearing, and he's going to have some problems, especially in that right ear. Anyway, one of the surgeons came down to see him and put him in the hospital for a couple of days. They used some vasodilators, and he regained blood flow in that foot, thankfully. Not sure about his hearing. But once again, Looper blew this guy off, and if he had done what Looper told him to, he would've lost that foot. He's either clueless or careless or both. Probably both."

This was a dangerous pattern, and I understood Brad's concern and frustration. If it had been happening in our hospital, I would first sit down with the surgeon and then with the chief of the surgical department. If that failed, there was the executive committee of the medical staff. But dealing with a physician at another hospital was problematic—something I'd never had to do.

"There are a couple more cases you need to know about—two people that Chuck Miller took care of."

Willis Abernathy was in the wrong place at the wrong time. He was at a remote tavern at two in the morning and had an unpleasant verbal exchange with another patron. This led to an altercation during which knives were drawn, and Willis was stabbed in the neck. His "friends" rushed him to the Divine Mission ER, dumped him on the sidewalk, and took off.

He had a stab wound just over his left clavicle, and after a quick assessment in the ER, Dr. Looper had been called in to evaluate it.

Willis's vital signs were stable, and he was alert, though still under the influence of several adult beverages. Looper listened to his lungs and heart, then asked for a surgical tray.

"We'll need to explore this wound and see how deep it goes," he explained to the wide-eyed Abernathy.

Without any local anesthesia, Looper probed the area with a blunt instrument, pronounced that it was superficial, and slapped a large Band-Aid over it.

"No chest X-ray, nothing," Brad huffed, shaking his head. "Just sent him home."

Willis had surfaced a few days later in our emergency department. Fever, shortness of breath, chest pain. Chuck Miller saw him, looked at the wound, and immediately ordered an X-ray. Willis's entire left chest was filled with fluid.

"Chuck thought it must be a hemothorax—that a vessel has been severed and filled his chest with blood. He put a chest tube in, and a yellowish fluid came out. No blood. One of the surgeons took him to the ER and found a lacerated thoracic duct with a chest full of lymph fluid. He'd never seen one before and didn't know if any of his partners had. Willis made it through the operation and went home after a week in the ICU. But that was close."

The thoracic duct drains lymph fluid from most of the body into a large vein in the left side of the neck. You have to go pretty deep to sever it, but that's what had happened to Willis Abernathy. Rare, but deadly. A Band-Aid wasn't going to fix it.

All of this was overwhelming, but Brad had one more patient to tell me about.

Charlie Hobbs was a painter and had been working at an industrial site. He was using a high-pressure paint gun, balancing on a ladder ten feet off the ground. He slipped on one of the rungs, and the gun fired into the palm of his left hand. He climbed off the ladder and went straight to First-Aid where the EMT on duty cleaned the small wound and put a dressing on it.

"Doesn't look too bad to me," the EMT told him. "But you might want to get a tetanus booster."

Charlie went to Divine Mission where he was given a tetanus shot. The wound was cleaned and examined, and once again, Dr. Looper was called to evaluate the injury. By this time, Charlie was in a good bit of pain and told Looper.

"Can't be that bad," Looper scoffed. "This is barely a scratch."

He directed the nurse to put some triple-antibiotic cream on the half-inch wound, followed by a bulky dressing.

"Keep it up in the air for a few days, and you'll be fine."

Chuck Miller saw him in our ER two days later. Charlie was in tears. His hand was swollen, red, and draining pus.

"Robert, a first-year intern is taught that a paint-gun injury is a real problem. The wound may be small, but paint is injected into the soft tissues at a high rate of speed. It has to be opened up and cleaned, or you're just asking for trouble. He should have been taken to the OR right away. Our hand surgeon first thought he might end up losing that hand, but he was able to save it. Lost all flexion in his fingers but can still move his thumb. Just another mishandled patient by Looper. When Chuck told me about this one, I had to do something. I knew I'd probably get into trouble, but I found out the name of the chief of staff over at Divine Mission, and I called him. I explained what we've been seeing, and he told me he would handle it. I hope this doesn't bounce back on you, but what could I do?"

Brad had done the right thing and gone through the proper channels. I needed to explain this to Stanley Baker. It might still bounce back on me, but sometimes doing the right thing comes with a price.

"Don't worry about that, Brad. This guy is dangerous, and someone needs to do something before another person is hurt. Thanks for telling me this."

"Stanley, let's talk about this surgeon down at Divine Mission. I think there are a few things you need to know."

The CEO was sitting behind the large desk in his office, thumbing through a stack of papers.

"Interesting that you brought that up, Robert. I just got off the phone with the administrator there. I was calling to apologize for the actions of Dr. Hayes, but it seems the problem has handled itself. One of the floor nurses reported to the administrator that she had gone into a treatment room last Saturday morning and found this Dr. Looper operating on himself."

"What?" I exclaimed, trying to picture what he had just said.

"Yep. Apparently, he had a ganglion cyst on the back of his left hand and had numbed up the area, scrubbed it with Beta-dine, and was in the process of cutting it out when she walked in the room. It must have surprised him because he started swearing at her and throwing things. Scared her to death. Don't know how he sewed up his hand. But when the administrator called Dr. Looper's office on the following Monday, he was told the office was closed and that Dr. Looper was no longer practicing. He was moving out of state somewhere."

This was all too much, and I tried to collect my thoughts. It didn't matter what state he was in, Francis Looper was going to be a danger to anyone who crossed his path. It couldn't stop here, and I would need to call our licensing board and get their advice. It had to be done.

"And you can counsel Dr. Hayes about the right way of handling things," Baker added, leaning back in his chair. "Remind him that it's important that we have a good relationship with Divine Mission, and that they continue to send us patients. Very important. Let him know that he's on my radar."

After I notified the state board, I'd be on his radar too.

The hard thing to do and the right thing to do are usually the same thing.

—Anonymous

Really?

When you've worked in the ER long enough, at some point nothing surprises you. Except when it does.

The ER—4:00 a.m.

Andy Rankin, one of the orthopedists on staff, shuffled down the hallway and plopped into one of the chairs behind the counter of the nurses' station. We had called him a few hours earlier to take care of an elderly woman with a fractured hip, and he was just now finishing up. In another chair sat our unit secretary, Amy Connors, and to her left was Jeff Ryan, the lone nurse on duty. We had done our share beating back disease and pestilence, and the department was now empty of patients.

"Took a while to fix Mrs. Weathers," Rankin said. "But she's fine now and should do well. Nice family."

The Weathers family *had* been nice—caring and supportive of their mother and grandmother, never leaving her side until she was rolled into the OR.

This was the time of day in the ER—the dark, sleep-deprived hours—that invited reminiscences, ruminations, and the occasional nostalgic recollections. I thought of the Weathers family and remembered another elderly patient—someone we had seen a few months ago.

"Andy, you up for an interesting story?" I asked him.

"I've got all night," he answered, glancing up at the large clock above the ambulance entrance. "What's left of it."

"You mentioned the Weathers family. Not too long ago, we had another family—great people also—who brought their grandmother to the department. She was 92 years old, and prior to this visit, had been clear as a bell. Walked two miles every day, didn't take any prescription medicine, and had a memory like an elephant. I guess that's a good thing. Anyway, she had some significant changes, and her two daughters and their children brought her in to be checked. One of the daughters told me that her mother was 'sundowning'— something she had recently read about and was sure her mother had.

"'Tell me about this,' I asked her. 'How did it manifest?'

"'Well, in the evening, she gets confused, almost delirious. That's something new, and we're worried.'

"'How new is this? When did it start?'

"The other daughter quickly spoke up. 'Just this evening. That's when it started.'

"That's mighty fast for the development of dementia. I assumed that must have been their concern with the sundowning, if indeed that's what it was. But there are a lot of causes for the acute onset of confusion that we would need to worry about.

"We were all over there in room 5—I pointed to the cubicle behind Andy Rankin—and for the first time I noticed a small dog wrapped up in a blanket and lying on the woman's belly. It was a Yorkie, I think. Anyway, it was small, and it was asleep.

"I asked the daughters about that, and one of them said, 'Momma won't go anywhere without Fru-fru. The doggie keeps her calm, and we didn't want to do anything to disturb her.'

"Momma was sleeping quietly herself and didn't appear to be disturbed by much of anything.

"Her vital signs were completely normal, as were all of her lab studies. Her cardiac exam was fine, and the only thing I could find was some mild lethargy. When I shook her shoulder and spoke close to her ear, she would open her eyes, roll them around in their sockets, and raise her right hand as if waving goodbye. All the while she was smiling—a sweet, peaceful, happy smile. Didn't make much sense. I told the family we would need a scan of her brain to make sure nothing bad was going on there.

"'Can Fru-fru go with her?' someone asked.

"'No, Fru-fru will need to stay with you. They won't allow her in the Radiology department.'

"Two of the X-ray techs walked into the room, and one of the daughters picked up the dog. Fru-fru rolled her head around, looking at everyone in the room, and struggled to get down. She was on a leash, and the daughter carefully put her on the floor.

"'What in the world?' a granddaughter remarked. 'She's never done anything like that before.'

"We all watched as Fru-fru took a few wobbly steps toward the entrance of the room, then spun in a full circle with her head pointed at the ceiling. She stopped dead still, reared back, and started howling. It was closer to a donkey's bray than a howl, though much higher in pitch, and I couldn't help but laugh. How could this small dog make such a sound? She dropped her head, rolled it around, and started spinning in circles—chasing her tail.

"'Well I never...' stammered a daughter. 'What's gotten into that dog?'

"We were all staring at the pup when a strange noise came from the stretcher. Grandma was starting to howl, and it sounded a lot like Fru-fru. She waved her arms over her head and was peacefully grinning, yet her eyes remained closed."

"What in the world, Robert!" Rankin remarked. "What was going on?"

"Well, I had my suspicions," I answered. "I looked around the room and noticed that everyone was staring wide-eyed, mouths hanging open. Everyone except one of the grandsons. He must have been about 14 or 15, and he stood with his back up against a wall, staring down at his feet. I needed to have a word with him, so I tapped him on the shoulder and motioned for him to follow me out into the hallway.

"We stepped into the room next door, and to his credit, the boy spilled the beans. Well, he spilled them after I bluffed him a little and told him I knew something was up, and he needed to come clean. He admitted that he and a couple of guys had been at a friend's house earlier in the day. The friend's parents were out of town, and they decided to make some *special* brownies. One of the guys brought some marijuana, but they had never done this before, and the recipe they used was...well, it was pretty strong. They each ate one and split up the rest. The grandson was supposed to have dinner at his grandmother's house and set the bag down and forgot about it. Apparently, Fru-fru found it, carried it to Grandma's room, nibbled on a little of it, and Grandma ate what was left. The rest is well…history."

"Really?" Andy Rankin said, shaking his head. "That's hard to believe."

"Believe it, Dr. Rankin," Jeff said. "I was here and heard that dog howling. Grandma too."

"And she did okay?" Rankin asked.

"She did fine," I told him. "We kept her overnight, and the next morning she was good as new. They're gonna have to keep the brownies away from her, but she was fine. So was the dog. She was fine too, except for her name. They could have done better than that."

Rankin chuckled. "That's pretty strange, but let me tell you about a case I had when I was a resident. I was rotating through Internal Medicine when it happened."

Andy was a second-year orthopedic resident in the program at Charlotte Memorial Hospital, and as part of his clinical exposure, he was spending a couple of months on an Internal Medicine rotation. A good bit of that time was spent in the ER, responding to a request from one of the emergency department physicians to help sort out a difficult or confusing problem. Some of these patients were figured out quickly with more extensive testing or imaging procedures. Some were never completely diagnosed, and the senior Internal Medicine residents, along with their attendings, just did the best they could. And some left everyone scratching their heads.

Bartholomew Evers was a professor of chemistry in a small college in the area. As if taken from the pages of a dusty eighteenth-century novel, he walked into the ER wearing brown wing-tipped shoes, olive corduroy pants, a blue cotton shirt covered by a knitted vest, and was bespectacled with black, horn-rimmed glasses so thick that his eyes appeared magnified more than twice their normal size. He had a pipe tucked into his vest pocket, and it was easy to imagine him sitting in a chair, puffing on that pipe, and studying some thick, ancient tome.

The ER doctor was the first to see Professor Evers and was confused by the constellation of his complaints. Sore mouth, swollen eyelids, swollen and tender gums, and swelling on both sides of his neck. He complained of a "metallic taste," but what had brought him to the ER this particular morning was persistent nausea and vomiting.

"Not sure what's causing this," he had told the doctor. "Thought maybe it was a virus and it would pass. But nothing seems to be helping the nausea. And now with my neck swelling, I wonder if I have the mumps."

The ER doctor latched onto this possibility and went back to the nurses' station to consult one of his medical texts. Scanning the pages that listed the symptoms, findings, and diagnosis of this childhood disease, he ruled against the possibility.

"Sandra," he said to the unit secretary, "put a call into whoever's on for internal medicine. We'll let them figure this out."

Andy Rankin followed the third-year internal medicine resident, Jackson Andrews, to the ER. Along with them was a family medicine intern, and she and Andy chatted about Clemson football, Tar Heel basketball, and the general state of ACC athletics.

Andrews walked over to the ER doctor and said, "Okay, where is this conundrum you have for us?"

With chart in hand, Andrews led the team into the room, where they found Bartholomew sitting quietly on a metal chair, legs crossed and arms folded in his lap. He looked up and nodded as they entered.

The senior resident led the questioning—probing the professor's medical history, work history, and anything that might offer some clue as to the cause of these symptoms. While not life-threatening, they posed a diagnostic dilemma, and that's what internists lived for.

After a thorough physical examination and a battery of lab studies, Andrews was left scratching his head. The swollen salivary glands caused him the most consternation. He had thought of mumps himself but ruled out that possibility. And there was no fever, no weight loss, no signs of a malignant process. He looked over at Andy and the family practice intern for their thoughts. They both rolled their eyes and looked at the ceiling.

Andrews took a deep breath and sighed.

"Well, Professor Evers, it seems..."

The exam room was located near the ambulance entrance, and the blare of an arriving rescue vehicle had startled the professor, causing him to sit bolt upright in his chair, head swiveling around the room.

The family medicine intern was the only one to notice, but Evers, while reacting to the loud blast, had reflexively raised his right hand to his shirt pocket. When he finally relaxed, he dropped his hand back to his lap.

She stepped toward him, tapped the front of his shirt, and asked what was in his pocket.

"We don't need to..." Andrews interjected, waving a hand at Evers.

"No problem," the professor said, reaching into his pocket and taking out a small medicine bottle. He handed it to the intern.

"Is that one of your prescription medications?" Andrews asked.

"No, this is one of my...It's an over-the-counter formulation."

"Potassium iodide, 130 mgs," the intern stated, studying the label on the bottle. "No directions. Looks like it's a supplement or something."

"Not a supplement, my dear," the professor gently instructed. "It's a preventive therapeutic."

"A what?" Andrews asked, reaching for the bottle.

Bartholomew Evers proceeded to explain his possession of this compound and how it was used. There was a nearby nuclear power plant, and the main risk of a disastrous accident would be the release of radioactive iodide—I-131.

"Just like Chernobyl," he explained to the enthralled group. "Clouds of the stuff fell on the whole area and on the people living there. An epidemic of thyroid cancer followed—still happening to this day."

The response to an exposure of I-131 is to take a dose of potassium iodide, and to take it as quickly as possible.

"If you take it within one hour of exposure, there's a ninety percent chance of preventing any problems, but if you wait as much as six hours, that drops to fifty percent. After twelve hours, well, there's no use in taking it."

He then went on to explain how concerned he was about such an exposure, and because quick action was called for, he would take a dose of the potassium iodide every time the power plant activated an area-wide siren alarm. It was designed to be a test of the system, a drill, and they had all heard it before—several times. It turned out that whenever Evers heard the siren, he would take a pill, and then do so daily for as much as a week—much more than the recommended dose. Over the past month or so, there had been several siren tests, and he had been taking the stuff daily for at least five weeks.

"Do you think this might be causing my problems?" he asked, pointing to the medicine bottle.

Andrews pulled a worn copy of the *Washington Manual*—his internal medicine resource bible—from his pocket and searched the topical index in the back. He flipped to the indicated page and quickly read the section titled "potassium iodide toxicity."

Bingo.

"What happened to that guy?" Jeff asked Andy. "Did all that stuff go away?"

"It did," Andy answered. "We saw him a few weeks later in follow-up, and everything had resolved. He swore that he would stop taking the potassium iodide unless there was a real emergency, and I hope that's been the case. But you never know. Good thing that family practice intern was there. We would probably have missed it. I know I would have."

"A chemistry professor," I mused. "You just never know."

We were all quiet for a moment, letting the story of the marijuana brownie and chemistry professor sink in. Then I remembered TJ Holmes.

"We need some help over here, Dr. Lesslie."

It was Lori Davidson, and she had just deposited a young man in room 4 and was helping him onto the stretcher.

I handed the chart I was working on to Amy and pointed to the orders section.

"Chest X-ray and CBC," I instructed her.

I walked over to room 4 and pulled the curtain closed behind me.

TJ Holmes was a 22-year-old college student, dressed neatly in khaki pants and a long-sleeved, blue, button-down shirt. He was wearing loafers but no socks.

He sat on the stretcher with his legs dangling beneath him and stared blankly at the wall in front of him.

"What's going on here?" I asked Lori.

TJ heard the question and mumbled, "Thash ovar twa ooo...ooo ma..."

He struggled with the last word, such as it was, and gave up.

"Can't make any sense out of what he's trying to say," Lori told me. "Some friends dropped him off outside of Triage and took off. The only ID we have is a Target card with a name on it—TJ Holmes—and he seems to respond to that."

"No help from his friends before they left?" I asked, hopeful but doubtful.

"Nope. They took off without a word. I didn't see any evidence of trauma out in Triage, but I have no idea why he's here— other than this obvious confusion. And he smells like somebody dumped a whole bottle of aftershave on him. Maybe Aqua Velva."

I hadn't heard that name in years. I leaned close, sniffed, and quickly recoiled.

"You might be right. It's some kind of cheap aftershave for sure."

TJ was confused, to be sure. Delirious and possibly delusional. We would need to be careful lest he suddenly became violent.

He remained calm while I examined him, looking for some subtle evidence of a head injury or bodily trauma. Nothing. His cardiac exam, other than a mildly elevated heart rate, was normal, as was the examination of his lungs. It was his neurological exam that concerned me.

Lori looked at me and said, "When those guys dropped him off, one of the techs led him into the department, and his gait was off. He was stumbling and almost fell. His balance was just about gone, and I got him in a wheelchair as fast as I could."

Confusion, gait disturbance, no evidence of trauma. A couple of red flags popped into my head. We would need to rule out some intracranial problem—a tumor or bleed, especially of the cerebellar area—or an overdose of some kind. With no medical history—or history of any kind—we had little to go on.

I ordered a battery of lab tests, drug screen, blood alcohol, and a CT of TJ's head. Hopefully, in all of this there would be an answer.

"Jaa whooo laaa nay," he mumbled.

I gave up trying to make sense of this garbled mess and left the room.

His labs came back completely normal, and a drug screen checking for everything we could showed only a small amount of marijuana—nothing that would explain his findings. While in the department, nothing changed. He remained calm, but sat staring at the wall, mumbling incoherently.

Finally, two radiology techs walked into his room to take him for his CT scan. I hoped that would be the answer, and that it would be something that could be fixed.

TJ and the two techs had just turned the corner at the end of the hallway when one of the hospital's groundskeepers walked up to me. It was the middle of July, and he was sweating, with blades of cut grass plastered to his forehead.

"Dr. Lesslie, somebody gave me this." He was holding a long, narrow, dark bottle, and he thrust it toward me. "Tapped me on the shoulder and almost threw this at me, then took off runnin'. Yelled something about takin' it inside to the doctor, and I guess he meant you."

He took a step backward, ready to get out of the department.

I stared at the bottle and without looking up said, "Thanks." *What in the world is this? And why was I supposed to get it?*

I looked up to ask another question, but he was gone.

"What you got there?" Amy Connors asked, eyeing the strange container in my hand. I placed it on top of the counter, and she slowly turned it, trying to see the label.

"Wormwood," she said. "It's the Green Fairy."

"What? How did you know that?" I asked, picking up the bottle and searching the label's whimsical writing.

"Absinthe," I murmured.

"That's right, absinthe," she echoed.

She reached behind her and grabbed a clear plastic cup from the lab cart.

"Here, pour a little into this."

The bottle was half-empty and corked. I easily removed the stopper and poured an inch of pale green liquid into the cup.

"Green Fairy," Amy said again. "Pretty, isn't it?"

It *was* pretty. I lifted the cup to my nose and sniffed.

"Whew! That's potent!"

The alcohol vapors were strong, and my eyes began to water.

"Mostly alcohol," she told me. "Supposed to be a hallucinogenic, but not so much. Mainly, it's the alcohol. Used to be you could only get it in Europe and had to smuggle it into the States. But now you can get it around here, even 'starter sets.'"

"Starter sets? How do you know so much about this?"

"Doc, I haven't been around every block, but I've been around a few of them."

I did some checking, and it turned out that everything Amy told me about absinthe was dead-on. Long thought to cause hallucinations, it was the alcohol content that addled the brain and not some mysterious, secret ingredient. If a person was suggestable—and most of us are—the cloudiness of ethanol can be perceived as the touted, mythical effects of this beverage. No hallucinations or delirium—just an old-fashioned buzz.

The radiologist called me with TJ's CT report while the young man was getting back onto his stretcher.

"Everything's fine, Robert. Nothing here. I hope you find an answer to this fella's problem."

"Thanks. I think I have."

"Oh," Amy said, sliding a slip of paper across the countertop. This is his blood alcohol report. The machine was down until a few minutes ago."

I scanned the paper. ETOH 357 mg/dL. Three times the legal limit. That explained a lot.

This time when I went into his room, TJ was sitting on the stretcher with his hands on his knees, calm and quiet. He looked at me as I entered and asked, "Where am I? What am I doing here?"

We watched him for a while longer, and then when he was sufficiently sobered, released him to his friends. They had miraculously reappeared after Lori called one of them with a number given her by TJ. He was walking as if nothing had happened and would be fine.

"I thought absinthe was supposed to make the heart grow fonder," Amy mused.

"No," Andy was quick to respond. "You're thinking of..." He stopped midsentence, having just caught the tail end of Amy's wink aimed in my direction.

"Really, Amy?" he said, shaking his head. "Really?"

> *Truth is stranger than fiction, because Fiction is obliged*
> *to stick to possibilities; Truth isn't.*
>
>   —Pudd'nhead Wilson (from Mark Twain)

14

Index of Suspicion

Sometimes the answer is right before your eyes—obvious and clear-cut. But first you need to know the question.

The ER—Friday, 2:45 p.m.

"Ouch, I bet that hurts."

I was standing in front of the X-ray view box, studying the films of a 52-year-old man who had been raking leaves, fallen, and injured his wrist.

Jeff Ryan was our Triage nurse this afternoon, and I hadn't seen him walk up behind me.

"Yeah," I agreed. The fractured radius was badly angulated and would need some work getting realigned. "Who's on for ortho?"

I walked back to Ortho to give Leonard Stevens the news. His wife, Gail, was sitting on the stretcher beside him and got up when I entered.

"Keep your seat," I told her. "I just want to tell you about Leonard's X-rays."

He looked familiar, but then a lot of people I see in the ER look familiar. I tried for a moment to remember where or when I had last seen him but gave up and focused on the task at hand.

"We're going to put a splint on that wrist and send you to one of the orthopedists' offices. They're expecting you and will get you in right away."

I handed his wife a copy of his X-rays and turned again to Leonard.

"Any questions?" I asked. He was standing close to me, and my mind made a fleeting note of the red, blotchy bumps clearly visible on his nose. Unusual for his age.

"Thanks, Doc," he answered, heading for the doorway. "Don't know how that happened, but I'll be more careful."

His wife gave me a strange look—her eyes narrowed, and her brow furrowed. Her mouth opened a little, as if she wanted to say something. Then they were gone.

"Frequent flyer," Amy Connors said, sliding a thick medical record across the counter to me. "Been here a lot."

I glanced at the name on the chart. "Leonard Stevens." The record was over an inch thick, indicating multiple ER visits and possible hospital admissions. That was a lot, and unusual for someone his age. He and his wife had left the department, and I had a bunch of patients to see. This would have to wait for another day

I slid the chart back to Amy. "Thanks, but we can return this to Medical Records."

Two weeks later, Leonard was back in the ER—this time with a sliced left thumb. He was helping his wife in the kitchen, dicing tomatoes, when the blade slipped, opening a two-inch gash.

No tendon or nerve involvement, but it would take a while to put him back together.

"Let's numb this up, and then you're going to need some sutures," I told him, drawing a local anesthetic into a syringe. "This will hurt for just a second, and then you won't feel anything more."

His hand trembled a little, but nothing unusual, considering what I was about to do.

I finished with the painful part of this procedure and was turning toward the doorway of Minor Trauma.

"Let's give this about ten minutes to take effect, then I'll be back."

"Dr. Lesslie," his wife quietly called to me.

"Gail," Leonard immediately uttered, his voice stern.

I turned and looked at Gail Stevens. Her eyes averted mine, and she looked down at the floor.

"It's starting to get numb already," he said. "Thanks."

I looked at his wife once more, then left the room.

"Well, look what the cat dragged in!"

Amy was looking over my shoulder, and I turned around to see Harriett Gray walking into the department through Triage.

"You're not a patient, are you?" Amy asked, smiling at her friend.

"No, no. Nothing like that. I'm just visiting."

She walked over and gave me a hug—a welcomed and comforting grandmother hug.

Harriett was in her early seventies and had retired from the ER four years earlier. She and Virginia Granger had trained in nursing school together, and after each going their separate ways, had reunited in the Rock Hill General ER, spending more than 15 years together.

Harriett was a favorite of every staff member who passed through our department. She was a rare and interesting combination of empathy, wisdom, and perceptiveness, coupled with a quick and nimble mind. She knew who was sick and who wasn't, and she knew when one of us—her "children"—needed a knowing word or a warm, nonjudgmental shoulder to lean on. She and Virginia appeared to be opposites—Harriett's warm and welcoming persona, and Virginia's apparent gruff, impenetrable exterior. But those differences were in appearance only. They were fast friends and an amazing team of two nurses—dedicated to our patients and to each other. And they both cared for the ER staff—their "family."

"Just visiting?" Virginia asked. She had been in her head nurse's office and heard the voice of her friend. She walked over to the nurses' station and joined us. "I bet we could find an extra uniform somewhere and put you to work."

"Too old for that," Harriett chuckled. Then she sighed and looked at her friend. "The real reason I came was...I need to talk with you, Virginia." Then she turned her head toward me. "You too, Dr. Lesslie."

"Sure, Harriett." A puzzled look spread across Virginia's face as she motioned for the two of us to follow her into her office.

"What have you done now?" Amy tossed in my direction.

I was puzzled as well, and once in Virginia's office, I closed the door behind me.

"I need to talk with you about Leonard Stevens," Harriett began. "Gail, his wife, is the best friend of my daughter, and she came to my house a few days ago in tears. She didn't know where else to turn."

She was talking about Leonard Stevens, the man back in trauma with the lacerated hand.

Harriett proceeded to tell us of Gail's concern for her husband and for his increasing use of alcohol. For years, it had been a problem for him, causing difficulties with his wife and family, and now most recently at his work, where he was the plant manager of a large manufacturing concern. Whenever the issue was addressed, he fell back into a resolute denial, blaming any problems on those around him. Lately, that blame had fallen largely on Gail, and she was nearing a breaking point. She had suggested counseling, either with their minister or with an expert in alcoholism. He had raged at the word and would have none of it.

"She's at her wit's end," Harriett sighed, shaking her head. "She called me when Leonard cut his thumb and told me they were headed here, to the ER." She paused and looked at me. "I was hoping you were on duty, and was thinking...hoping that you might be able to talk with him. To at least get him to begin to see that he has a problem."

It wasn't the first time she had brought an issue like this to my attention. Sometimes it was a strained relationship among members of the ER staff, or the occasional but much-needed pulling up of my own bootstraps. But this would be tricky.

Those odd bits of information suddenly fell into place. The skin changes of his nose—sometimes associated with heavy alcohol use—his thick medical record, his wife trying to tell me something but being cut off. These were all red flags, and I should have paid attention.

"Who's his family doctor?" I asked her.

"Willard Rogers," she answered.

Virginia grunted and shook her head.

"Didn't he just retire?" I asked Harriett.

"Getting ready to," Virginial grumbled. "End of this month, but none too soon."

Willard Rogers was an elderly family practitioner who lived in a nearby town. He had been in the area a long time and still had a lot of patients in Rock Hill. He was cheerful and friendly enough, and when I first came to Rock Hill, he was still seeing his patients in the ER. He was never without his worn and clichéd black bag, and never without a large and flamboyant bow tie. He also carried a silver-tipped walking cane, something he never used except as part of the image he wanted to present—a carefully manufactured image. I had gone behind him enough and seen enough of his patients to know that the care he was giving was less than acceptable. Wrong medications, wrong dosages, wrong diagnoses. None of us are perfect, but as a physician, Rogers set a new standard of incompetence. Worse still were the contents of his medical bag. He had left it at the bedside of a patient he was seeing in the ER, and I happened to glance at it in passing. His stethoscope, such as it was, was hanging from one side. Its tubing was worn and cracked, and I wondered if anything could be heard through it. Lying beneath it were two small, silver flasks. One was full, and the other half empty. As he left the department that evening, I caught a whiff of alcohol as he passed by. When I talked with the chief of the medical staff a few days later, expressing my concerns regarding Dr. Rogers, he told me that the administration was aware of the problem, but that it had handled itself. Rogers was resigning from the active medical staff and would no longer be seeing patients in the hospital. That would fix part of the problem, but the larger one—his actively seeing patients in his office—seemed to be beyond our reach.

"What about his office practice?" I had asked. "He has a real problem, and his patients are at risk."

"There are channels to deal with that, Robert. And the administration will be pursuing them. If you learn of any more specific problems, let me know."

That was troubling. But the *most* troubling reality was that his patients trusted him. In fact, they loved him. It's sad but true that many of our best physicians seemingly have little personality, and because of that are not held in high regard. The opposite of that is the more troubling. You can fool some of the people some of the time... Go figure.

"Not going to be any help there," I said, disappointed that Leonard Stevens was still seeing Willard Rogers. Another physician might have been able to confront Leonard in an honest, forceful fashion—something that was sometimes needed, but that required judicious timing and commitment born of caring. I couldn't envision Rogers doing that.

"Let me see what I can do."

Leonard Stevens's old records were sitting on the countertop of the nurses' station. It had been a little more than ten minutes since I had left him and his wife, but he should be fine. I needed to take a look at his history.

Flipping through the record, I saw my own handwriting. He had come to the ER a couple of years ago with a back strain. Nothing serious, and I had sent him home with something for pain and some stretching exercises.

There were other ER visits. Shingles, a bad headache, the flu, a sprained ankle and twisted knee. Seemed like a lot.

The next part of the chart contained detailed reports from a hospital admission only four months ago. *Strange, he hadn't told me about that.*

The discharge diagnosis was "pneumonia" and the treating physician was...Willard Rogers. Stevens had been in the hospital for almost a week—a long time for a straightforward pneumonia in a reasonably healthy individual.

The discharge summary, dictated by Rogers, was sparse and of little help. I turned the pages to his lab studies, scanning through the myriad values, looking for something out of line, something that might give me some guidance.

Normal. All his chemistries were fine, including his blood sugar and electrolytes. Liver studies were normal as well—

something that would have pointed to any damage caused by excessive alcohol intact.

His CBC was...

I was running my finger down the list of values—white count was a little high, platelets were normal, hemoglobin was fine. When my finger reached the "indices" part of the report, I stopped. These numbers, these "red cell indices," gave us information about the size of his red cells and the amount of hemoglobin contained in each cell. In the face of excessive alcohol intake and a frequently associated vitamin deficiency, the cells become large and pale. Leonard's indices were abnormal—some of the worst I had seen. It should have grabbed Rogers's attention and caused him to ask some questions. But he had probably focused only on the white cell count and hemoglobin, if he had looked at them at all.

This was enough information with which to confront Leonard Stevens and impress upon him the damage that his drinking was doing. *Good luck,* I told myself.

I turned toward Minor Trauma just in time to see Leonard exit the hallway bathroom and walk toward Minor. His movement caught my attention and caused me to stop where I stood and watch. He was shuffling a little, but it was there. When he walked directly away from me, his gait was broad based, planting his feet shoulder width apart and focusing intently on maintaining his balance. It could be a sign of a cerebellar disorder, one cause of which was excessive alcohol. That was another piece of information, but it would have to be handled carefully.

Leonard didn't feel anything while I sutured his thumb and

rested quietly on the stretcher with his eyes closed. It took a little more than half an hour to put the gaping wound back together, and since he was a captive audience, I was able to broach the topic of his alcohol use.

"You're bleeding pretty good," I remarked, though it was not really excessive. "Do you take baby aspirin?"

He shook his head.

"How about alcohol? It can cause some bleeding problems."

Gail's head turned in my direction, then back to her husband.

"Aw, maybe a couple now and then," he answered. "Nothing out of the ordinary."

I stopped suturing and held my hands in the air.

"What's the ordinary?" I probed.

He was losing patience, but he finally admitted that he was drinking around three or four beverages a day. Every day.

His eyes were still closed, and I glanced at Gail. She slowly raised an index finger and pointed it at the ceiling.

I was running out of sutures to put in, and he had reached the limit of this line of discussion. I tried to impress upon him the importance of limiting his drinking and explained how it was showing up in his blood work.

"Dr. Rogers never said anything about that," he responded defensively. I was finished, and he sat up on the stretcher. "I'll go by and see him before he retires and see what he has to say."

I shared my observation of the way he was walking, and he blew it off.

"My leg fell asleep, that's all."

They walked through the doorway and headed toward the

exit. He was moving slowly, carefully placing one foot in front of the other, obviously determined to prove me wrong. Gail turned and mouthed, "Thank you." And then they were gone.

Harriett Granger was standing in Virginia's doorway, watching as the couple left.

"How did that go?" she asked. "Were you able to bring up his drinking?"

"I was," I told her, shaking my head. "Not sure any of it sank in though, but it might be a start. I just wish he had someone he could talk to— someone he respected and that might be able to talk some sense into him. He's got some problems, subtle now, but they'll only get worse."

"Well, Dr. Lesslie," Harriett sighed, "thanks for trying. I'll give Gail a call later this evening and see what she thinks. You know, you're right. If there was someone who would shoot straight with him, that might be a start. I've even thought about my husband sitting down with him. They know each other, but..."

She stopped, and her gaze dropped to the floor. Virginia stood behind her. When our eyes met, she slowly shook her head.

"Thanks again, Dr. Lesslie," Virginia said, putting an arm around her friend's shoulders. "I'm going to walk Harriett out to the parking lot and will be right back."

A few weeks passed. I had occasionally thought about the Stevenses and wondered if Leonard had gotten some help. It bothered me that no one—including me—had put together what was right in front of us. If we had paid attention to these subtle details or asked the right questions...but I needed to stop beating myself up. We had taken care of his broken wrist and put his lacerated thumb back together. And I had taken care not to lay some heavy guilt trip on him. I had done what I was supposed to do.

One morning, when he was once again on my mind, Virginia walked up to the nurses' station. I was about to ask about him when she said, "I guess you heard about Leonard Stevens."

That's almost always an introduction to bad news, and I cringed.

"No, tell me."

Gail had called Harriett just a few days ago and told her that Leonard was doing better. A lot better. He had seen another doctor in town and was trying to stop drinking. AA was being considered, but he wasn't quite ready to take that step. Yet, he was trying, and Gail was hopeful.

The next evening, Leonard Stevens was killed in a single-car accident. It's never too late...until it is.

> *Discernment is God's calling to intercession, never to faultfinding.*
>
> —Corrie ten Boom

15

On Holy Ground

The ER—Thursday, 2:30 p.m.

I was standing beside Lori Davidson at the nurses' station, going over the things that needed to be done for our patient in Observation.

"Dr. Lesslie, do you have a minute?"

It was Virginia Granger. And she wasn't smiling.

Lori looked at me, picked up the chart we were working on, and walked away.

What had I done now?

I followed Virginia into her office, closed the door behind me, and sat down in a chair across the desk from her.

"Heard you had a difficult case yesterday. A two-year-old with an ethylene glycol ingestion. Good work," she said, not looking up from a report in her hands.

"You can thank Denton Roberts for that one," I told her, wondering what she was so intently reading. Denton had been the paramedic responding to the scene of an unresponsive child. He had noticed an open container of ethylene glycol carelessly left on the floor of the garage and had astutely made the connection. We were ready with the proper antidote when the child arrived in the ER and were able to quickly turn things around. "Denton's really sharp and figured that one out."

"Uh-huh," she murmured, distracted by something.

She dropped the papers to the desk and looked up at me.

"It's Harriett Gray," she said somberly.

My heart sank.

"I noticed she was acting a little...off the other day," I remembered. "What's the matter with her?"

"It's not Harriett. It's her husband, Stu."

I had met Stuart Gray—Stu, as he insisted—years ago during one of our many ER gatherings. He and Harriett were always there, even after she retired. This past Christmas, he had pulled me aside after my unjustly much-booed act in our "talent show."

"Robert," he began, his eyes searching mine, "how are you handling the stress? I know what goes on in the ER, and I know it can take a toll."

This was no passing comment or superficial question. Stu always cut to the chase, and I thought for a moment before responding.

We talked a while about the things that really bothered me—abused and neglected children, abused seniors, the needless harm we inflicted on each other, and the most haunting: those people who I wanted to save but couldn't. These were the things that always elicited a strong and painful gut reaction.

"It's not your *gut*," he had said. "It's your heart. And you have to keep it."

Keep my heart? What did that mean?

"Heart work," he said, sensing my struggle. "It's the hardest thing we can do, but the most important. A few hundred years ago, John Flavel wrote that 'the greatest difficulty in conversion—coming to Christ—is to win the heart *to* God, and the greatest difficulty after conversion is to keep the heart *with* God.' Think about it. A lot of truth there, and if you can keep your heart *with* God, the things of this earth seem much less important. We'll be able to handle the bad stuff that comes our way, and that includes what you deal with in the ER."

Maybe that was Stu's secret. Heart work. He was one of those people who seem to radiate peace and a palpable sense of calm, assurance, and wisdom. He brightened every room he entered.

"What's going on with Stu?" I asked Virginia.

"Eight months ago he was diagnosed with pancreatic cancer," she said quietly.

We both knew what that meant. It's a bad disease, and few people survived it.

"He's been seeing one of the oncologists here in town and tried chemo, but nothing has worked. He's stopped all of that."

"I didn't know," I told her.

"No, they wanted to keep it quiet. Just family members and a few close friends at their church. Nobody here knows about it."

I could understand that. And now I understood Harriett's reaction the other day when she mentioned her husband.

"She wanted to tell you about Stu," Virginia said. "But I think it was too much for her in that moment."

We were silent. Virginia rubbed her hands together, and I stared at a pen on her desktop.

She sighed and looked up at me. "He's in hospice now."

I nodded. That would be a good thing, considering his diagnosis and the fact that he had decided to stop treatments. Once that decision is made, the more time he has in hospice the better.

"The hospice team has been a real blessing, especially for Harriett," she said. "The nurses are something special, but so are the social worker, chaplain, and the aides that come once a day. They've all been able to help with a lot of things and given her a lot of support and advice. And they've kept on top of his pain. Of course, that's important, to him *and* to Harriett."

I nodded again and remained silent.

"I think you know his hospice nurse, Julie Childers."

"Julie? I didn't know she was doing hospice work now."

Julie Childers had been a nurse in the ER until three years ago. She was great at what she did, and I was always glad to have her working with me. A year before she left the ER, her 11-year-old son died with leukemia. It was a long, difficult death, and Julie showed the strain and heartache. We didn't think she would come back to work in the ER, but she did. When young children came in with an emergency, she was always the first to help them, the first to be at their side. And when we lost a young one, she wanted to be the one to sit with the family, to console them as best she could. She had been there.

"I know I'll never get over losing Jamie," she had once told me. "But if I can help someone through this kind of grief and pain, even in some small way, I want to try."

Maybe that was why she was a hospice nurse now. She's walked the walk.

"Yes," Virginia answered. "She's been with one of the local hospices for a couple of years now. I just found out when I saw her at Harriett's."

"Hmm," I murmured, then fell silent again. This was a lot. Harriett had a piece of my heart, and Stu was a special guy. "I'm really sorry about that."

Virginia placed both palms on her desk and leaned toward me.

"Stu wants you to come by the house. He wants to talk with you."

"When?" I asked her.

"What are you doing when your shift ends?"

Virginia tapped lightly on the front door. We heard footsteps approaching, and I took a deep breath. The door opened, and there stood Julie Childers. She saw me, grinned and gave me a bear hug.

"How long has it been?" she asked. "Two, three years?"

"Too long," I answered. "It's great to see you."

Virginia barged past us into the house. "Come on. You two can catch up later."

I hadn't known what to expect, what the home of a dying man would look and feel like—even smell like. I've been around a lot of death, probably too much, but it was usually in the ER. It was an environment that I controlled, and it almost always involved strangers—people I had never met. This was different. I knew Harriett and Stu Gray, and I knew this was going to be hard.

The front door closed behind me, and I was immediately struck by the light. Sunshine poured into the foyer and beyond, making the home come alive. The smell of fresh-cut flowers wafted over me, and Harriett appeared. Without a word, she walked over and put her arms around me. Deep, painful sobs welled up from within her, and she trembled. I felt her tears on my neck, and my own streaming down my face. I loved this woman, and I loved her husband.

"Okay, that's enough," she said, stepping back and keeping both hands on my shoulders. "Let's go see Stu."

I was about to wipe my eyes with a shirtsleeve, when out of nowhere Harriett handed me a box of Kleenex. I thanked her, dabbed my eyes, took a deep breath, and followed her down the hallway to their bedroom. Julie and Virginia walked behind.

The door was half-closed, and Harriett flung it open. Once more, sunlight flooded the room, brightening every corner, every inch. On one side of the room, a small writing table groaned with stacks of books, piled high and spilling onto the floor.

Stu was reading, propped up in the bed by three or four pillows. A brightly colored plaid blanket was drawn up to his waist. His bedside table was littered with an assortment of pill bottles, a box of Kleenex, a half-full glass of water, and a much-worn Bible.

He dropped the book to his chest and looked up at us. Then his eyes focused on me.

"No time for tears," he smiled. He had seen my eyes, still red and swollen.

"Hello, Virginia," he said cheerfully. "Thanks for coming by, and thanks for bringing Dr. Lesslie."

"I didn't have to ask him twice," she said, still standing in the doorway, smiling.

"Okay, you two skedaddle," he said weakly, motioning Virginia and Harriett out of the room with the back of his hand.

The door closed, and now he motioned to me.

"Have a seat, Robert, and pull that chair a little closer."

He was pointing to a small, leather-covered and comfortable-looking club chair, and I did as instructed.

He settled back on the pillows and straightened his blanket.

Just as I hadn't known what to expect when I entered this home, I didn't know what to expect when I would see Stu. It had been several months since we had seen each other, and I knew the ravages of this cancer would be taking their toll.

He was dying. The muscles and veins of his neck strained beneath taut, pale skin, and his cheekbones protruded, casting shadows over his gaunt cheeks. He was wasting away, slowly disappearing.

But his eyes were alive with a piercing light. They captured mine, and for a moment I forgot his disease-ridden body lying before me.

"So, I bet you wonder why I asked you to come over," he started with a grin. "I know it's not the place you want to be spending your time. Heck, it's not the place *I* want to be spending *my* time. But here I am."

I nodded and leaned closer, my forearms resting on my thighs.

Stu took a deep breath, and I heard a faint rattle. He cleared his throat a couple of times and began.

"Robert, I learned a long time ago to listen to that all-important still, quiet voice. Not my conscience, mind you. That will only confuse and mislead me because it comes from our emotions or the echoes of our deepest desires, both of which distort what's real, what's true. It took me a long time to hear that voice and to tune in to it. You remember us talking about 'heart work'? Well, this is part of that work, tuning in to that voice like you would a violin. When it's tuned, you hear beautiful music, but when it's off, even a little, it's…well, it's not so lovely. And when it's way out of tune, it's awful, and you might not hear anything except a screeching that makes your skin crawl, and you finally stop listening at all." He paused and studied my eyes. "Any of that make sense?"

I nodded. It was the voice of the Holy Spirit. While not always successful, I tried to listen for it and to pay attention. But life too often drowns it out.

"Good. Then you'll understand when I say that this quiet voice kept whispering to me, telling me that I should talk with Robert Lesslie. Didn't know what about, only that I should talk with you. I figured once you were here, I'd know why."

He folded his hands behind his head and nestled into the pillows.

"So, I want to share some things with you—some things that have been on my heart."

I leaned back in my chair, waiting for him to continue. In that moment, there was nothing in the world but the two of us, surrounded by stillness and a comforting peace.

"We pay too little attention to our spiritual lives, too little time sorting out the things that are really important. That's been true for me. We get lost in what someone has called the 'wilderness of trifles.' That's a good description, isn't it? We focus on the trifles of our lives, the things that decay and pass away and that have no real meaning. That's part of our heart work—to search for the trifles in our life and to get rid of them. Not easy —that's why it's called *work*. One of those trifles is that we spend too much time dwelling on our physical needs—money, prestige, clothes, even food—and not enough time on our spiritual needs."

He paused and took another deep breath, gathering his strength.

"I'm afraid that if we fed our bodies like we do our hearts, we'd starve. Our basic human nature is one of being out of balance. Here's a question for you."

He dropped his hands to his lap, and I leaned a little closer.

"What was on your mind when you first awoke this morning? Something occupied your thoughts. What was it?"

I struggled with this question, trying to remember. I daresay it had nothing to do with Stu's "heart work. "

"That's always a tip-off as to the state of our spiritual life. What's the first thing we think about in the morning? Then we need to consider the last thoughts we have before falling asleep. Those things tell us a lot, and they're things we can control. But it takes..." He paused, raised his eyebrows, and stared intently at me.

"Work," I answered. I was paying attention.

"Work," he echoed, smiling. He reached for the glass of water at his bedside and took a sip. He was visibly tiring but determined to continue.

"I've had a lot of insights during my life, Robert. *Epiphanies* some might call them. I believe they're glimpses of truth, reminders of important spiritual matters. One of those came to me during the early morning of my sixty-ninth birthday. That was eight years ago, long before this stuff started," he paused briefly, waving a wasted hand in the direction of his medication bottles.

"I was reading James Montgomery Boice. It was his study on the book of John. He repeatedly made the point, taken from the very words of Jesus, that Christ was God Himself, made flesh to walk among us, and that it was God Himself on that cross. You may already understand that, Robert, but when this reality worked its way into my heart, it was something new, something I had not fully understood before. And I wept. Jesus is not some vague concept, some hard-to-grasp mystical figure. He is God Himself, and it was the love of God that we nailed to that cross. He suffered there willingly for us. For you and for me. I don't pretend to understand everything. I still see 'through a glass darkly,' as Paul tells us. But one day, and it won't be long for me, I will see clearly. What a day that will be!"

Stu took a deep breath, and there was that rattle again. He closed his eyes. This effort had exhausted him.

The door opened behind me, and Julie walked into the room. "Okay, Mr. Gray," she announced. "It's time for your nine o'clock meds." She caught my eye and nodded. "Past time."

Stu opened his eyes, their brightness dimmed by his fatigue.

"Fine, Julie," he said quietly, struggling to sit up.

I got out of the chair and bent over him, putting my hand on his weak, bony shoulder.

"Thanks, Stu."

A thousand thoughts flooded my heart—things I wanted to say to this man. But sometimes words aren't enough—sometimes words aren't needed.

I gently squeezed his shoulder and again whispered, "Thanks."

He nodded and smiled.

I stepped into the doorway and stopped, not wanting to leave this room, this special place.

And then I heard his voice one last time.

"Remember to keep that violin tuned."

I never saw Stu again. Virginia told me he passed a few days after my visit—peacefully, without pain.

"Harriett wanted me there with her," she told me. "Their two sons were with them, along with their wives and children. It was the middle of the afternoon, and Stu had wanted the curtains opened. Sunlight flooded the room, and somehow seemed to shine directly on his bed. We sang one of his favorite hymns, and then his son had a prayer. Stu said goodbye to everyone there and closed his eyes. His breathing just sort of...slowed. After a few minutes, he whispered, 'It is well,' and he was gone."

Tears filled her eyes. "I wish you could have been there with us. The Lord was in that room, holding Stu...holding each one of us. That moment was...it was..."

"Holy."

> *Then the Lord said to him, "Take off your sandals, for the place where you are standing is holy ground"* (Acts 7:33).

16

Every Hundred Years

The ER—Tuesday, 2:30 p.m.—a week before Christmas

We need a lavage tray over here! Stat!"

Ross Collins stood in the doorway of Major Trauma, calling out to anyone who would listen.

"Coming," Lori Davidson responded. She gave me a questioning glance as she hurried past me.

Collins had joined one of the family practice groups a few months ago, right after finishing his residency. He was bright, friendly, and at least for now, would come to the ER to see his patients.

He had one in Major Trauma—a three-year-old boy whose mother had called, telling him she had found Freddie chewing on some poinsettia leaves.

"The green ones or the red ones?" Collins had asked her.

"I...I don't remember," she stammered. "Red, maybe..."

"Okay, just get him to the ER right away. I'm in the hospital and will meet you there."

I was in Ortho when the child came in. Collins was waiting and pointed the mother into Major Trauma.

Now he was in the hallway again, calling for a lavage tray. It was needed to wash out the stomach of someone with a serious ingestion, but only if it was indicated, and only if we had to. It was no fun for those on either end of the large, plastic tube.

A moment later, Lori appeared in the doorway of Major. She anxiously nodded her head, motioning me to the room.

Freddie Withers was sitting quietly on the stretcher wearing only some Batman underwear and staring wild-eyed around the room. His mother stood beside him, pale and biting the knuckles of one of her hands.

"Oh, hi, Dr. Lesslie," Collins said, looking over as I walked toward the stretcher.

"What do you have?" I asked, my eyes flitting from the boy to his mother and back to the doctor.

"Poisonous ingestion," he responded. "Poinsettia leaves."

"You need some help?"

"No, but thanks anyway. I can handle it. I'll just need to get his stomach pumped out and probably admit him to the ICU. He seems stable right now, but you never know."

A quiet gasp escaped from Freddie's mother. Lori stepped over and put a hand on her shoulder.

"Poinsettia leaves?" I asked Collins. I leaned closer to the boy and saw a faint, red rash around his mouth.

"Yeah, they had a couple of plants in the house, and Freddie got hold of some leaves and maybe ate a couple. Mother doesn't know if they were red or green."

Red or green? What did it matter?

One of the ER techs bolted into the room carrying a blue, paper-wrapped tray. In bold letters written on its top was the word *Lavage*. She handed it to Lori and backed away from the stretcher.

Lori held the tray in both hands and looked at me with raised eyebrows.

Before I could react, Collins took it from her hands, dropped it to the countertop behind the stretcher, and ripped it open.

The contents of the tray were sparse and in plain view. A stack of sterile gauze, some lubricating jelly, a "bite-block," and an evil-looking plastic coiled tube. The tube was clear, three-quarters of an inch in diameter, and about three feet long.

"I need some gloves, nurse," he said over his shoulder. "Size seven."

Freddie's mother was watching all of this and intently studying the tube.

"Does that thing..." she whispered.

"Ross," I said, interrupting his preparations. "Hold on just a second."

He spun around and faced me. "What?"

"I'm not sure this is really necessary," I began gently, prepared to voice a more insistent objection if that failed.

"What do you mean?" he asked, snapping a glove onto an outstretched hand. "Poinsettia leaves are extremely toxic, especially the red ones. And we don't know which ones he ate. It hasn't been that long ago, and we need to empty out his stomach."

I would have preferred to have this conversation out in the hallway, away from Freddie's mother, but Collins was charging ahead.

"Poinsettia leaves," I began again, "or any part of the plant can cause some minor symptoms but no real problems. Mainly skin irritation, like you see around his mouth. And maybe some mild stomach upset, but nothing serious. The best treatment is to rinse out his mouth, wash off his face, and observe him for a couple of hours if you want."

"Not toxic?" he uttered in apparent disbelief. "But I've always heard that..."

"Old wives' tale," I said quietly. "All of the toxicology literature is in agreement."

An audible sigh escaped from Freddie's mother.

Lori covered the lavage tray with the torn wrapping, hiding the tube from view.

"Are you sure?" he asked, his brow furrowed.

I nodded and didn't move.

"Okay then," he sighed. "This is your area of expertise, and I'll trust you, Dr. Lesslie. Nurse, can you help the boy rinse out his mouth and wash off his face?"

Freddie remained in the department with us for two more hours, and when our staff could no longer keep him from running around the department, we sent him and his mother home.

Later that shift, Ross returned to the ER and pulled me aside.

"Dr. Lesslie, listen...uh...I just want to thank you for helping me out with that child this morning. I had just always heard that..."

"It's okay," I reassured him. "I know you've just finished your residency, but now comes the hard part: putting it all together—what you've learned, and what's practical. We all have to do that when we start out. I know I did."

He nodded, thanked me again, and walked out of the department.

Ross Collins was well intentioned and bright, and with enough experience and some seasoned mentoring, he would be fine. The important thing was that he was open to being mentored and accepted it without headstrong resistance.

A week later, Lori Davidson was standing beside Collins while he was making some notes on the chart of one of his patients. He said something to her, nodded, and walked back to the ENT room.

I had just come on duty and seen but not heard this exchange.

"What's going on?" I asked her.

"Oh, nothing," she responded. "Just helping Dr. Collins with a patient."

She picked up a chart, walked over to room 2, then disappeared behind its curtain.

"*That's* a good nurse."

I turned around to see Saul Geller standing behind me. He must have slipped into the department through Triage, and I hadn't noticed him.

"You're right about that," I agreed.

Saul was in his late sixties—one year away from retirement. Well, he had been "one year away" for the past six or seven years, but each time his retirement was mentioned, it seemed the entire hospital staff tried to talk him out of it. He was the head of the maintenance department and had been for more than 30 years.

He stood before me in his customary attire: blue denim work pants, a light-blue, long-sleeved shirt stained with several obligatory grease smears, and wearing a tired leather tool belt, replete with a dangling set of at least fifty keys, two screwdrivers, a tape measure, and a dangerous-looking box cutter. He was a little overweight, balding, and wore thick, black glasses that might have obscured the profound intellect and wisdom behind them. If you knew Saul, you soon learned to never doubt his intellect or his wisdom.

Saul Geller knew every inch of Rock Hill General. He was on the staff when the hospital was being built, and during its construction, he crawled through every nook and cranny in the expansive structure. When something mechanical went awry, he was usually the first to respond and always the one to correct the problem. To some, he might be an unsung hero, but to those of us who depended on his expertise, he was the real deal—a true hero when we needed one.

I had learned a few years ago that Saul was also an excellent chess player, successfully competing around the state and winning an impressive number of tournaments. It made sense. He was very analytical in his approach to whatever problem we might throw at him: electrical, plumbing, heating and air. It didn't matter.

"You know, that doctor's going to be a good one too." He nodded in the direction of Ross Collins. "Young, but he's going to be okay."

I didn't doubt that but was curious about Saul's perspective.

"Tell me what you mean," I asked him.

"Well, I've seen him around the hospital—in the ER and up on the floors. And I've seen how he interacts with his patients and their families. And how he treats the nurses and staff. That tells you a lot about someone. He's always calm and friendly and wants to know what's on someone's mind. Then he takes the time to listen—something a lot of you folks in your white lab coats don't often do." He chuckled and watched for my reaction.

"Hmm," I muttered. "I can't hear you. I'm not listening."

He chuckled again and continued. "I have a good friend who was having some prostate problems a few months ago. Had an elevated PSA, and we were worried about cancer. A couple of us talked him into seeing one of the urologists in town, and he had some biopsies done. Turned out to be a low-grade malignancy and something that could be handled with surgery. While that was being scheduled, he started having chills and fever and felt miserable. They told him it was a prostate infection and put him on some antibiotics. Didn't get any better, and one morning I was mentioning this to Ella Hughes, the head nurse up on 3-B. Dr. Collins was sitting nearby and overheard what I was telling her. He told me to bring my friend by his office and let him take a look. Turns out it wasn't a prostate infection after all. It was an infection of one of his heart valves—endocarditis, I think he called it. When he had the biopsies done, apparently some bacteria got loose in his bloodstream and settled on one of those valves. Anyway, it was still early and not much damage had been done. But had Dr. Collins not caught it, the bacteria would have chewed up that valve, and my friend would have been in trouble. He's fine now and had his prostate surgery. Cancer free."

"That was a good pickup," I said and meant it. Diagnosing endocarditis is not easy. The symptoms are subtle, the associated fever comes and goes, and your index of suspicion has to be high. You have to think about it, or you'll miss it.

"Yeah, Collins's going to be fine," Saul said thoughtfully. "Still counting the steps."

"Counting the steps?" I asked him, struggling to make sense of his metaphor.

"I read a lot of C.S. Lewis," Saul answered, studying me. "Lewis has a lot of interesting and important things to say. One of those had to do with learning to dance, and he was relating it to our spiritual lives and how we learn to worship. Anyway, he said something like 'as long as you notice and have to count the steps, you're not yet dancing—only learning to dance.' That applies to a lot of things. I know it applies to what I do around here. Took me a lot of years to learn how to dance. And I'm sure it applies to becoming a good doctor. You have to count the steps and figure it out until it becomes natural. Then you're dancing."

He paused and slowly nodded his head. "Dr. Collins is still counting his steps, but he'll get there. He'll be dancing."

A few months after this conversation, Saul Geller was once again in the department—this time as a patient lying on the stretcher in our Cardiac room. He had walked up to Lori David-son and told her he was having some unusual chest pain. Within minutes, he was in Cardiac with an IV taped to his arm, O2 prongs in his nostrils, and an EKG streaming out of its machine.

It showed the cause of his chest pain: Saul was in the middle of a heart attack, and he wasn't doing well.

Once I saw the EKG, we started an IV infusion of a "clot buster" and waited for evidence of the opening up of his coronary vessels. It didn't happen, and I watched nervously as his blood pressure hovered just above a dangerous level.

Dr. Eldridge, one of our cardiologists, had examined Saul, looked at his EKG, and walked out of the room to the nurses' station. I followed him.

"What do you think?" I asked. "No response to the thrombolytic, and his pressure bothers me. I asked Lori to call the cath lab and let them know we would probably be sending him over."

"That's what we'll need to do," he agreed.

Amy Connors dropped some lab slips on the countertop, and Eldridge reached for them.

"Hmm...looks like his diabetes is not well controlled."

"Diabetes?" I was surprised by this comment. Saul had denied any medical problems, and he was on no prescription medications. "He's not a diabetic," I said to Eldridge.

He slid the report toward me, and I immediately saw the glucose level: 385 mg/dl.

"What?" I muttered.

"That would explain the lack of response to the medication you tried. If he's had poorly controlled—or noncontrolled—diabetes, he could have small vessel disease, making everything worse. We won't know until I can see his arteries, and I hope there is something we can do, but it might be difficult."

"Difficult?" I stammered. My friendship for this man was overtaking my clinical reasoning.

"There may be *nothing* we can do," Eldridge said matter-of-factly. "We'll just have to see."

I walked back to Cardiac and stood by Saul's side. He was pale, and his skin was clammy.

Lori looked up at me. "Cath lab will be ready for him in five."

"Good." I turned to Saul and said, "You told me you don't take any medications, right? No history of diabetes or any medical problems?"

"Right," he answered quietly.

"Your blood sugar is sky-high," I told him. "No way of telling how long that's been going on. When's the last time you saw your family doctor?"

He sighed and played with an edge of the hospital sheet.

"Saul?" I prodded.

"Well, I don't have a family doctor. I just come down here if I'm sick or something. Otherwise, I don't bother."

Amazing. Here was a man of considerable intelligence, a man who paid minute attention to the inner workings of this hospital, and who totally neglected the inner workings of his own body. Now he was in trouble.

"Dr. Lesslie, is it all right if Saul has a visitor?"

Amy Connors stood in the doorway. Behind her I could see a middle-aged man, peering into the room over her shoulder. Saul's wife had died a little more than five years earlier, and I knew he had two sons who lived within an hour or so of Rock Hill. This must be one of them.

"Sure," I said. "But he'll be heading to the cath lab in a few minutes."

The man walked into the room and directly over to Saul. He took his right hand in both of his and held it, not moving, not saying anything.

Saul looked up and smiled. "Roy, what are you doing here? You ought to be working."

"They can spare me for a little while, Saul. I heard you were having...you were here, and I wanted to check on you. The boys can make do for a little while."

Boys?

Saul looked at me and said, "Doc, this is Roy Stillman. He runs the Boys' Home here in town. Has been for...how many years?"

Stillman shook his head. "A long time, and with a lot of your help. But don't worry about that now. You just..."

"They're ready in the cath lab!" Amy shouted from behind the nurses' station.

Lori unlocked the stretcher's wheels and rolled it toward the doorway.

Saul looked up at me, smiled, and said, "Every hundred years."

"What?" I was scurrying beside the stretcher, trying to keep up with Lori.

"Every hundred years," he repeated. "Ask Roy."

They hurried through the doorway and out of sight.

Roy Stillman and I stood in the Cardiac room alone.

"I didn't know Saul was involved with the Boy's Home," I said.

"Involved? He was much more than that. After his wife died, that's where he spent most of his time, when he wasn't working here at the hospital. When we needed money for some unforeseen expense, he was there. When we needed help or one of the counselors was sick, he was there. The boys love him. We all love him. I wanted to be here for him for a change."

That all made sense. Saul Geller was a selfless individual, always ready to jump in and help where he could.

"What's this about 'every hundred years'?" I asked.

Roy chuckled. "That's something he would frequently say to the staff, and to the boys as well, when they would listen. The whole thought went, 'Every hundred years, all new people.' His point was that after that number of years passed, maybe a few more, the world would be inhabited by all new people. Everyone here today would be gone. It was a challenge to address our own mortality—the fact that we are only passing through—and to learn from the past, hope in the future, but live in the present. Today—this day. That's all we really have."

He paused and looked at me.

"Every hundred years," I quietly repeated. "That's an interesting thought."

"It is, isn't it? And an interesting perspective. Some might find it a little depressing if this world is all that we have, and we're just passing through. Not Saul. In fact, he finds comfort in the thought. He's convinced that while this world will one day disappear, what we do here—today—the lives we touch, that's important. 'Roy,' he used to say, 'this work that you're about is important, and you need to take it seriously. You need to take the time you're given seriously because it matters. What you're called to do matters. Just don't ever take yourself too seriously,' I've tried to live by those words. I know Saul has."

Roy had given me a lot to think about. And Saul...suddenly it struck me. Saul was telling us something. "Every hundred years..."

Roy Stillman disappeared through the ambulance entrance, and I walked over to the nurses' station.

"I can tell you're worried about Saul," Amy sighed. "And that makes me worry."

I took a deep breath, sighed, and felt a chill course through my body.

The hospital intercom erupted overhead, and we stared at each other.

"Code Blue, cath lab! Code Blue, cath lab!

Every hundred years.

> *My prayer is that when I die, all of hell rejoices that I am out of the fight.*
> —C.S. Lewis

17

"Houston, We Have a Problem"

M ike Brothers reached from the backseat and handed the taxi driver a $20 bill.

"Keep the change, Hasan." He had read the driver's name displayed on the dash, and whenever he could, he tried to call people by their name.

Hasan responded with a nod and a smile.

Sharon had already gotten out of the cab and was standing on the curb, waiting on her husband. Mike slid across the seat and joined her. They both looked up at the towering, glassed building in front of them and read the bold lettering high above.

MD Anderson Cancer Center

"This is a big place," Mike sighed.

The front passenger window of the cab opened, and Hasan leaned toward them.

"Mr. Brothers," he called.

They both turned and looked at the driver.

"You will have a miracle before you leave Houston."

He waved as the window rolled up, then pulled into the early morning traffic and disappeared.

Rock Hill—three months earlier

"What's the matter, Mike?" Sharon asked.

They were leaving church and were almost to their pickup truck. Sharon had noticed Mike fidgeting in their pew, occasionally placing a hand on his stomach. He was walking slowly now, and his color had a greenish hue.

"It's my stomach," he muttered. "Must have been something I ate at the fish camp last night."

The hospital's EMS team had met at one of the local restaurants the evening before, and since Mike and Sharon had been emergency responders for more than 20 years, they had wanted to attend. "Crash," as Sharon had been nicknamed, provided most of the entertainment—mainly just by being there.

"You sure?" she asked. "We ate the same stuff, and I feel fine. Do you think we need to get it checked out?"

"Nah. I just need to get home and lie down for a while. It'll pass."

It didn't pass, and by six o'clock, Mike was in significant pain. He changed his mind about being checked out, and they headed for the Riverview Medical Center—the local urgent care facility. The doctors there had worked in the Rock Hill General Emergency Department and had known Mike and Sharon for years. For the past few years, Sharon worked there part-time as the scheduling nurse.

"Well, Mike, I don't think it's your appendix," Sam Chase reassured them. The young doctor leaned against the counter of one of the exam rooms and flipped through the lab slips attached to Mike's chart. "White count's up a little, but nothing serious. Your urine is fine, other than some sugar from your diabetes, and your abdominal X-rays look good to me."

"That's a relief, Dr. Chase," Sharon said. "I was gettin' worried about appendicitis. But what do you think is causing the pain? It's not getting any better."

"You can say that again," Mike groaned.

"I can't say for sure," Chase answered. "And I'm concerned about the amount of pain you're having. Your belly is soft, and I don't think anything surgical is going on. But I don't want to send you home until we have a better idea of what's causing the pain. We'll need to send you to the hospital in Pineville to be seen in their ER and to get a CT scan of your abdomen. Just to be sure."

Mike looked down at his watch. It was a little after eight. "Well, there goes the night," he sighed.

"Don't you worry about that," Sharon scolded. "This is important, and Dr. Chase, we appreciate your help. Should we head up right now?"

The Pineville hospital was 30 minutes away—more than enough time to notify the ER staff that Mike would be coming and what they had found with his workup.

"Yes," Chase answered. "You two head out, and we'll get in touch with the ER. And don't eat or drink anything."

"See, I told you," Sharon lectured. "NPO. Nothing by mouth...or nothing oral...or...whatever."

Mike shook his head. His color was still green, and he muttered, "That's not gonna be a problem."

When they arrived in the Pineville ER, Mike's pain had almost disappeared.

Sharon had been driving and looked over at her husband. "Okay, let's go."

She opened her door and was about to get out when Mike laid a hand on her arm.

"I'm a lot better now, honey. Let's just head on home. We don't need to waste any more time. I'm fine."

His color was better, but she was still worried.

"Nope. Get out of the car, and we're going to get you looked at."

There would be no arguing with her. Mike took a deep breath, opened his door, and followed her to the ER entrance.

The staff was expecting them, and they were quickly led to one of the exam rooms. Mike's vital signs were taken, more lab work was done, and he was sent to Radiology for an abdominal CT scan.

"Everything looks okay," the ER doctor told them an hour and a half later. "Just like they found at Riverview, your white counts a little high, but that could just be from the pain you've been having. No appendicitis or kidney stone, and no evidence of an obstruction or any definite cause for your pain. That's the good news. The bad news is that I can't tell you what caused it. If you're still feeling all right, I think it will be safe to send you home and have your family doctor see you in a couple of days. Or you can come back here if the pain returns."

"I feel fine, Doc. Thanks for taking a look at me."

"Can we get a copy of all of his stuff?" Sharon asked. "The lab work and CT scan, just to give to our doctor?"

"Got it right here," the doctor answered, handing her a sheaf of papers. "And have them call us if there are any questions about what we found."

Mike jumped down from the stretcher and was in the doorway when the ER doctor added, "The CT scan didn't show anything going on in your abdomen, but the radiologist did note a couple of small nodules in the lower lungs. Wouldn't be causing any pain, but just let your doctor know. He might want to follow up on that."

"Sure, doctor. And thanks again," Mike answered.

It was a little after three in the morning, and they were both exhausted. Happy to be headed home and with no more pain, the words *small nodules* had not registered with either Mike or Sharon. The 45-minute drive home seemed to last forever, and once in their house, they collapsed in their bed.

After only two hours of sleep, Sharon was on her way to work at the Riverview Clinic. She stopped at a red light and glanced down at the hospital reports left in the passenger seat. The top page was the report of the CT scan. She glanced through the document and came to the bottom of the sheet where she found the words:

> IMPRESSION: Multiple pulmonary nodules as noted above. Rule out a metastatic disease.

The driver behind her began blowing his horn, startling Sharon. She glanced up and saw that the traffic light was now green. The horn blew again, and she felt her face flush.

"Hold your horses!" she huffed. She started through the intersection then decided to turn into the parking lot of a small convenience store. The driver sped by, blowing his horn once more.

Sharon gave him a glowering glance then reached over and picked up the CT report.

Pulmonary nodules? Metastatic disease? This couldn't be Mike's report. The ER doctor...

She remembered the doctor's parting comments—words that hadn't fully registered when they were leaving the ER—and wondered how they had missed them. She dropped the report and headed for the clinic.

At the nurses' station, she found Jim Kelly, the doctor on duty.

"Dr. Kelly," she addressed him, her face still flushed, but no longer from the obnoxious driver. "Could you look at this for me? It's Mike's CT report from the hospital in Pineville."

"How's Mike doing?" Kelly asked. "Dr. Chase told me you came in last night. He was worried about the pain Mike was having."

"That's gotten better," Sharon said, sliding the CT report in front of him. "I just need to know what to make of this."

Kelly studied the paper. He took a deep breath and turned to Sharon. "Did you and Mike know about this? Has he had a recent chest X-ray or any lung problems?"

"No. Nothing like that. He's never smoked or had asthma or any lung trouble. What do you think this means?"

"It might not be anything."

The hesitancy and tone of his voice betrayed his concern, and Sharon studied his eyes.

"But we'll need to work this up. The next step will be a CT of his chest with contrast. Just to be sure."

Sharon picked up the reports and turned toward her office. "I'll get on that right now."

When working in the clinic as the scheduling nurse, she made the arrangements for all radiology studies as well as physician referrals. She knew who to call and within minutes had Mike scheduled for the study that afternoon.

"I'm gonna do what?" Mike questioned over the phone. "I feel fine, and I don't need another CT scan. I've got to be at work in a couple of hours, so that's not going to happen."

He had been married to Sharon for too many years to think he would be able to talk her out of this and was already deciding who he would call to cover his shift.

"Mike…" Sharon drawled.

"Okay," he murmured. "Where do I go and when?"

In the past, I've shared with my readers that sometimes it seems we find ourselves standing on the platform of a train station. We're holding a ticket—no destination, just a blanket ticket to somewhere, anywhere. Then one day we get that ticket punched. It might be a routine doctor's visit, and our healthcare provider notices a small lump or a peculiar skin lesion. It might be some lab work that's a little off, or an X-ray that reveals a faint shadow, or the recent onset of a cough or other mild symptom that catches their attention. The ticket gets punched, and we find ourselves on a journey that leads to more testing or examinations. One step leads to another, and eventually our destination becomes clear. Often, it's a simple outcome—the train is leading us to a nonthreatening station and to a problem that can be easily resolved and is then gone. At other times, the destination is something we never dreamed possible—something dark and life-altering. Sometimes life-ending.

Without him even knowing, Mike Brothers's ticket had been punched.

Mike had the CT scan done in a facility in Rock Hill. It took only a little over an hour and a half, and he was back at work.

Sharon sat at her desk, talking with a patient about a gallbladder ultrasound report.

"It looks like Dr. Kelly was right. You've got some gallstones and some inflammation of your gallbladder. We'll need to arrange for you to see one of the surgeons here in town."

The fax machine on the corner of her desk beeped and clicked, and a report started printing. The woman on the phone was asking some questions, and Sharon tried to help while at the same time scanning the report. It was Mike's chest CT.

The phone almost dropped from her trembling hands, and she muttered, "I'll...I'll get back with you in...in..." She dropped the receiver to the desk and stared at the piece of paper.

REASON FOR EXAM: LUNG NODULES

IMPRESSION:

Multiple bilateral pulmonary nodules highly concerning for metastatic disease. PET scan recommended for further evaluation. Left lower lobe nodule, although small, would be amenable to percutaneous biopsy.

Sharon got up from her desk and walked out into the hall-way. One of the clinic nurses, Jerry Reaves, was standing nearby, and Sharon motioned for him to follow her into the Observation room. Once inside, Sharon closed the door and handed him the report.

"Tell me what you think this means," she said to Jerry, her voice trembling.

He scanned through the single page and came to the bottom, carefully reading the "impression."

Shaking his head, he looked up at Sharon and said, "This isn't good. Who is it?"

Sharon couldn't answer, and when Jerry saw the tears streaming down her cheeks, he looked again at the report.

Brothers, Mike BD 06/11/1949

He looked up again at Sharon. "This isn't...this can't be Mike?"

Sharon sobbed and nodded her head. She slumped onto the hospital bed, and Jerry sat beside her, putting an arm around her shoulders.

"When did this..."

"I've got to call him," she interrupted. "He has to know."

She started to get up, but Jerry held her more closely.

"I've got his number," he said gently. "Let me call him, and you stay put. Would it be best for him to come over here? And Dr. Kelly needs to know. He can give you two some direction and help you decide on the next steps."

Sharon nodded without really hearing. Her mind was

spinning, considering all of the possible outcomes—none of which were good.

"Sit tight, and I'll be right back," Jerry told her.

Mike was cleaning the back of his ambulance when he got the call to come to the clinic.

"Is everything okay?" he asked Jerry. "Is something wrong with Sharon?"

"She's fine, Mike. It's best that you just come on as quickly as you can."

No more discussion—just "come to the clinic." Within minutes Mike was on his way. His first thoughts were of Sharon. *Had there been some kind of accident? Was she sick?* He was only a few minutes away when he remembered the CT scan. They hadn't heard anything yet, and if the report had come in...

That must be it. The CT report was back, and it wasn't good. If it had been fine, Jerry would have told me. Or Sharon would have called.

He pulled into the clinic parking lot, found a space, and turned off the motor of his pickup truck. He sat there for a moment, studying the backs of his hands. They were steady and still. No hint of trembling. He realized his breathing was slow and measured, and he was calm. Strange, but he was calm. He glanced at the dash and saw the handwritten note he placed there a few days ago. He found himself frequently asking, "Why me?" when he came upon a passage in Isaiah that had spoken directly to him:

> Who has understood the mind of the LORD, or
> instructed him as his counselor? Whom did the LORD

> consult to enlighten him, and who taught him the right
> way? Who was it that taught him knowledge or showed
> him the path of understanding? (Isaiah 40:13-14).

He had the words memorized now, and they comforted him.
No more did he ask, "Why me?" Now he simply thought, "Why
not me?"

Jerry met him at the nurses' station and without a word led
him to Observation. Sharon was sitting on the bed. She was making every effort to be strong—to stop her tears. When Mike came
through the doorway, her hands flew to her face, and her sobs—
loud and painful—shattered the stillness of the room.

He stepped toward the bed and knelt before his wife. Taking her hands in his, he said, "Whatever this is, whatever kind of
problem I have, God's got this. I'll be fine. God's got this."

Sharon stood and pulled Mike to his feet. They stood in the
middle of the room, hugging each other and not saying a word.

The door opened, and Jim Kelly walked in. Jerry had given
him Mike's CT report, and Kelly waved it in the air.

"Okay," he said, mustering as much enthusiasm and optimism
as he could. "We've got work to do."

The next step in Mike's journey was to see a lung specialist.
The best pulmonologist in the area was in Charlotte, but when
asked for an appointment, Sharon was told it would be at least
four weeks.

She was sitting at her desk in the clinic when Jerry dropped in and asked about the latest developments.

"We really want to see this specialist in Charlotte, but he's booked up. I don't know who else to try, or if..."

Her phone rang. It was the pulmonologist's secretary, telling Sharon that there had been a cancellation in the schedule, and Mike could be seen tomorrow—if that was okay.

"Of course it's okay!" Sharon exclaimed. "We'll be there."

"See," Jerry said. "Things have a way of working out."

The lung specialist saw Mike the next day and ordered a PET scan of his chest. This would give them a better idea of what they were dealing with and the nature of these nodules.

The report from that study read: "Bilateral hypermetabolic lower lobe pulmonary nodules consistent with bilateral broncho-genic carcinomas." Cancer. It was what they most feared.

"This scan helps us," the specialist told them. "But in order to treat this, we have to know exactly what we're dealing with. We need to have some cells to study."

"A biopsy?" Sharon asked. Mike sat silently by her side.

"Yes, a needle biopsy. Not a dangerous procedure, and there shouldn't be much pain. But we need to get some of this tissue."

A week later, Mike was admitted to the Presbyterian Hospital in Charlotte for the biopsy. Sharon sat outside the treatment room as the procedure was taking place. She closed her eyes and prayed, trying to block out the disturbing thoughts that hovered and threatened her peace.

The sounds of hurried footsteps startled her, and she looked up to see two nurses bolting into the treatment room. She jumped up and followed them.

"What's wrong? What's the matter?"

Mike's blood pressure had spiked, and he was short of breath. One of the nurses led Sharon back out into the hallway and sat with her for what seemed like hours.

The surgeon came out of the room and walked over to Sharon. "Your husband is fine. His blood pressure got a little high, but it's normal now. And his breathing is fine—no pneumothorax or any problem like that. We'll watch him overnight, then he should be able to go home in the morning."

Sharon was relieved. But when she walked into the room, her relief turned to alarm. Mike was pale and downcast—far different from her cheerful and energetic husband.

"Well, that's done," he sighed. "I hope we're finished with this kind of stuff."

They weren't. The biopsy report came back as "inconclusive." The surgeon had retrieved some of the tissue, but the hospital pathologist was unable to make a definitive diagnosis.

"I'm sorry," the surgeon began. "But, Mike, you're going to need an operation. We're going to need to do a wedge resection of that right lung and get more tissue."

"Can't we just cut all of this out?" Mike asked, knowing the answer.

"I'm afraid that would be impossible" came the response.

The procedure was scheduled for the following week. Seven days of worry, anxiety, and fear.

"Maybe it will be nothing," Mike said one evening. "Maybe it's just some scar tissue or something."

Sharon didn't respond. They both knew better.

At every step of this journey, Mike and Sharon had family, friends, church members, and coworkers praying for them. They would both say—then and now—that it was comforting, reassuring, and needed. But those nights before the surgery were dark and sleepless.

A thoracotomy is not a simple or painless procedure. A long incision is made on one side of the chest between two ribs. These are then separated—pried apart—allowing for the surgeon to access the part of the lung that needs to be removed. The lung doesn't have nerve endings, but those muscles and soft tissue do. And it hurts.

The next morning, Mike was still under the influence of some heavy-duty pain medicine when the surgeon walked into his hospital room. Sharon sat by his side and looked up as he entered.

"Your husband's vital signs have been good, and there's been no fever," he began. "His blood sugar is up, but with his diabetes and stress of the surgery, that's to be expected. How do you think he's doing?"

"As long as he has the pain medicine, he's able to rest. But his chest really…"

She paused and looked at her husband. His eyes were closed, and she glanced back at the surgeon.

In a hushed voice she asked, "Have you heard anything from the pathologist? Any word there?"

The surgeon cleared his throat and rubbed his hands together.

"Yes, we have. And it's not what we expected. It's not what any of us expected."

He stopped and took a deep breath. Sharon stood and walked toward him.

"What did you..." she whispered. "What did they find?"

"Mike has...malignant melanoma. A very aggressive type. We didn't expect..."

"Melanoma?" Sharon uttered in disbelief. "How could that possibly..."

She stumbled backwards to her chair and slumped into it. She had enough of a medical background to understand what this diagnosis would mean. Melanoma was a killer. And it was in Mike's lungs—in multiple places.

"Does he have any history of melanoma?" the surgeon asked. "Or any family history?"

"No, I don't think so." Sharon's brain was in a cloud, and she was having trouble collecting her thoughts. "He's never...wait a minute. Thirteen years ago he went to see his family doctor with a sinus infection. While he was in the office, he asked him to look at a mole on his right shoulder, and the doctor didn't like the looks of it. He removed it, and it turned out to be a melanoma. He saw an oncologist and had biopsies of four or five lymph nodes, but everything came back negative. He's been to see him every six months without fail. And he's never had a problem."

"It's a tough disease," the surgeon said quietly, stroking his chin. "And that's probably where it came from. Now that we know what we've got, we'll need to get him in the right hands and hope for the best."

Hope for the best. Tears welled in Sharon's eyes as the surgeon closed the door behind him.

Mike had been resting quietly during all of this, his eyes closed. Sharon sensed movement on the bed and looked over to see Mike's head turned toward her, his eyes wide open.

"Don't worry, honey. God's got this."

The next train stop was in the office of an oncologist, Dr. Travis Brooks—a man who would become not only their guiding physician, but a close friend.

"Well, here's the plan," he began as Mike and Sharon sat in his office. "Surgery is not an option with this cancer. We're going to be using some fairly new drugs—immunotherapy—that will attack these lesions by boosting your own immune system and targeting the cancer cells. They've been effective in melanoma cases, and we'll hope they work here."

"Have they worked with stage IV melanoma?" Mike asked him. "That's what I've got, I think. Metastatic melanoma, stage IV."

"You're right, Mike. It is stage IV. And the results with this type of...Let's just say this will give us our best chance."

Sharon heard the hesitation in Brooks's voice and looked into his eyes.

"When you say best chance, just what..."

"Dr. Brooks," Mike interrupted her, "let's just say we didn't do anything. No treatments or immunotherapy or anything. How long would I have?"

Dr. Brooks slowly tapped his fingers on the desktop. After a deep breath, he looked directly at Mike and said, "Six months. If you're lucky."

Sharon gasped and slumped in her chair. Mike sat straight upright, nodded his head, and smiled. "Okay then, when do we start?"

The treatment schedule would be aggressive. The two drugs would be given by IV every three weeks for a year, with each infusion session lasting about four hours. Eighteen treatments total. PET scans would be scheduled at regular intervals to monitor the effects of the treatment.

Mike's first treatment was "like a breeze." The infusion took a little more than four hours, and then he was home. He felt fine, except for some fatigue, which he noticed after a couple of days. Three weeks later, he was in the oncologist's office, ready for treatment number two.

"I'm sorry, Mike," Dr. Brooks said. "Your liver enzymes are elevated—a known side effect of these drugs—and with your fatigue, I think we'll need to wait a couple of weeks. We're going to give you a course of prednisone. That should help any inflammation in your liver and will probably help your fatigue."

"Dr. Brooks," Sharon interjected. "Remember, Mike's a diabetic. When he's taken prednisone in the past, his blood sugar has gone crazy."

"I've had that in mind, Sharon. But I think the benefits will outweigh the risks. We need to cool off his liver and continue with his treatments. Just monitor his blood sugar, and let me know if it gets too high." Turning to Mike, he asked, "You've never been on insulin before, have you?"

"Nope. Always controlled it with diet and oral medication. I don't have any desire to be on the needle."

Brooks chuckled. "I understand. Just watch your carbs and your blood sugar. And drink lots of water. Let's see where we are in a couple of weeks."

Mike's blood sugars bounced around on the prednisone, but he was able to keep it reasonably under control. And he was feeling better. Less fatigue, and the prednisone was giving him more energy. Three weeks later, his liver enzymes had not returned to normal, and Dr. Brooks postponed treatment once again. Finally, after another three weeks, his lab work was stable, and Dr. Brooks gave the okay. Another four hours for the infusion. By this time, Mike and Sharon had become favorites of the entire staff, and during those four hours, everyone in the clinic managed to stop by his recliner and check on the two of them.

One of the staff members overheard Mike calling his wife "Crash," and they asked Sharon where that had come from.

"You just never mind," she huffed, her face red and getting redder.

"No, Sharon," Mike said. "They should know about that, and if you won't tell them, I will."

"Well, you're just going to have to be the one, 'cause I got nothin' to say."

She plopped down in a chair and folded her arms across her chest.

By this time, Mike had an audience of five or six staff members, including Dr. Brooks.

"This all began about 20 years ago," Mike started. "And yes, it was a dark and stormy night."

Sharon was an EMT, responding with her paramedic partner to a serious collision on Highway 5. It was a little after midnight, and a heavy rain was just beginning to ease up. A pickup truck had run through a stop sign and clipped the back end of a small Honda, causing it to spin into a nearby ditch. The two men in the Honda were employees at the Duke Power Catawba nuclear plant and were on their way home to Kings Mountain. The driver had lacerations of his forehead and left arm, but nothing worse than that. The passenger had a dislocated elbow, but no other obvious injuries. The car was totaled, and the two men wanted to be transported to the hospital in Kings Mountain.

"Fine by us," Sharon told them.

Her partner, Jim, was placing the passenger's injured elbow in a sling and helping him up into the back of the ambulance.

"Jim," Sharon called to him. "I know the way to that hospital, so you stay in the back with these guys. Should only be 25 or 30 minutes."

She had only driven this ambulance once before, and that was in the parking lot of the EMS substation. Still, how difficult could it be? You flipped on the engine's battery and cranked up the motor. Simple as that.

She took off down the highway, lights flashing and siren

blaring, waking every horse and cow within a mile or so. Sharon slowed the ambulance as they entered the city limits of Kings Mountain and headed toward the hospital down a four-lane boulevard, lined with lampposts that gracefully arched over the street. Their light reflected off the rain-soaked asphalt like diamonds, and Sharon thought what a pretty...

Something was wrong. The engine of the ambulance started sputtering, and the steering wheel lurched uncontrollably. She gripped it with all of her strength, trying desperately to keep the ambulance on the highway.

Bam! Bam! Bam!

She took out three lampposts before she could bring the ambulance to a stop. Then, one by one, the lights of a dozen posts in both directions went out.

"What's going on?" Jim asked, appearing in the small opening that led to the back of the ambulance.

Flustered, Sharon unbuckled her seat belt and shifted to the passenger seat.

"Here, you drive."

It turned out that with this particular model of ambulance, there were *two* battery switches that needed to be flipped in order to properly operate the vehicle. She had been given this instruction, but had overlooked the second switch, and the motor was freezing up just as they entered the city.

"No harm, no foul," her supervisor would later say. "Those two men from Duke were fine, and they appreciated your help. Wait, there is the matter of the lampposts."

It didn't take long for this tale to work its way through the entire EMS team—and beyond. No one is sure who first called her "Crash," but it stuck. In fact, the minister and most members of her church still refer to her as Crash.

"Now that's a story," Dr. Brooks laughed. "I think we've got a new name for you."

Sharon—oops...I mean Crash—tightened her arms across her chest and glowered at Mike.

Two days after the second infusion, Mike began to itch. First, it was the back of his neck, and then his arms. Within hours he was itching everywhere, and a red, angry rash was spreading over his entire body. Sharon gave him some Benadryl to try, but it didn't faze the itching. Nor did cold showers or any lotion they could find in their medicine cabinet. After two sleepless nights, Sharon called Dr. Brooks. He instructed them to come to the office as soon as possible.

"This is a known reaction to the medications," Brooks explained, examining the rash and shaking his head. "Though this is the worst I've seen. It's not really an allergic reaction. That's why the Benadryl didn't help. But a high-dose course of prednisone should improve the rash and help the itching. If the skin starts to break down, we could be looking at treatment in a burn center."

"A burn center?" Sharon exclaimed. Her head was spinning as she tried to understand what was happening.

Mike remained calm. He nodded and said, "How much prednisone do you want me to take?"

This time it would be 80 mgs a day—a large dose. And this

time his blood sugars skyrocketed. He tried to eliminate his carbohydrate intake as much as possible, to the point where one day he told Sharon, "I'm going out in the woods and live on roots and tree bark. Maybe that will help."

In spite of their best efforts, his blood sugars remained out of control, and he was started on insulin. His weight had dropped by 38 pounds, he couldn't sleep, and the itching persisted. He was miserable. Hovering over them was the fact that they had no idea where the cancer was. They had missed several treatments and had not had a scan of any type since this all began.

"Sharon, I feel like I'm climbing a mountain and keep sliding backwards. I'm just not getting anywhere. I'm tired and just want to stop. No more meds, no more treatments, no more doctors."

Sharon shared his frustration, but she wasn't ready to give up.

"I know you're tired, Mike. But I've talked with Dr. Brooks about a second opinion, and he is fine with that. You and I are going to Houston in three days to see the doctors at the MD Anderson Cancer Center."

She was out of the room before he could respond. While she was packing, the words of Isaiah echoed in his mind, and he once again found peace. Three days later, they were in an airplane, headed for Houston.

The cab driver taking them from the airport to their hotel was talkative and wanted to know what they would be doing in Houston. Sharon explained the nature of their mission, and the driver asked if he could pray for them.

"Sure," she answered. "But please keep your eyes open."

When they got out of the cab and walked toward the hotel, Sharon asked Mike, "Did you hear what he said?"

"Yeah. Something about a miracle."

The staff of MD Anderson was professional and friendly. Sharon had never met a stranger, so she and Mike were made to feel like family members. The visit with the team of oncologists lasted a couple of hours, with the various specialists going through all of Mike's records, taking a lengthy and detailed history, and examining his body. Especially the rash.

"I agree with Dr. Brooks," one of them remarked. "This might be the worst skin reaction I've seen to these particular medications. Yet, it might mean that the drugs are working. We'll have to see."

Lab studies and scans were scheduled for the next day, and they would meet once again the following day to go over the results and come up with a plan.

"I know Dr. Brooks has explained how serious this is," the lead oncologist said. "Stage IV melanoma is a…challenging problem. And you've had several complications. But we'll be looking at every possible alternative. You can be sure of that."

All the tests were completed by late afternoon, and Sharon and Mike had a little time to find a restaurant near their hotel. They had been told to expect a phone call the following afternoon—a Wednesday—to set up an appointment.

Late Wednesday morning, they decided to visit a nearby mall and kill some time wandering around. A little after one o'clock, Mike excused himself and looked for the nearest restroom. A few minutes later, he came out and walked toward Sharon. Tears were streaming down his face, and he couldn't speak.

"What's the matter?" Sharon said, hurrying toward her husband.

He shook his head and held up his cell phone.

"You got a call from the hospital?" she asked, knowing and fearing the answer.

He nodded. Through his sobs and tears, he managed to say, "It's gone! The cancer is gone!"

Sharon almost collapsed. The two of them sat down on a nearby bench.

"Tell me what they said!" she insisted. "They said it's gone?"

"Yes," he said, his voice husky with emotion. "No more treatments, no more drugs, no more nothing. They said to have a good trip back to Rock Hill."

"Give me that phone," she said, reaching out and taking it from her husband.

She looked at the most recent number and dialed it. Within minutes, she was talking to one of the oncologists.

"That's right, Mrs. Brothers. Your husband's lab work is fine, except for the elevated blood sugar we knew about. And all of his scans are normal. There's no evidence of cancer anywhere. And those lesions in his lungs—they're gone. Nothing but scar tissue. We've never seen this kind of response with only two rounds of treatment, but it's happened here. Mike will not need anything further—no more immunotherapy or anything like that. He *will* need close monitoring, and we'll be setting up a series of scans in three months. I hope that sounds okay."

"It's more than okay! If you were standing in front of me, I'd hug your neck!" She thought for a moment and added, "So this is a remission."

"No, it's not a remission. His cancer is gone."

Gone.

Neither of them can remember the next few hours. Months of fear and physical suffering, and now to be told Mike was free of cancer!

"I told you God's got this," Mike reminded her.

"Of course He does," she agreed. "He always has. But we'll need to stay on top of this and do our part. We'll need to be back here in three months."

The next morning they were packed and headed for the airport. As they walked through the hotel lobby, someone called their names.

"Mike, Sharon!"

It was Hasan, their taxi driver. He was carrying the luggage of a couple who were just checking in.

"Hey, I know you got your miracle," he called to them across the packed lobby. "God is good!"

God *is* good.

Three months later, Mike's scans were completely clear. No evidence of cancer. And all the ones following that have been clear. After almost four years, he remains cancer free. He and Sharon know that they're still on that train, and they don't know where it will lead. But the one thing they do know, the thing that brings them courage and peace is that "God's got this."

One Sunday morning, the minister of Mike's church asked

him to speak to the congregation and to share his experiences. The following Wednesday, he and Sharon were in the fellowship hall with many of their church family. Mike referred to some notes he had made and told those gathered the story you've just read. Then he put his notes away, took a deep breath, looked around the room at his family and friends—those people who had been praying for him for so many months—and he began.

"Throughout all of this, God has never left me. He's carried me the whole time, and He had a plan for me. I had no idea what that plan would be—I'd never have chosen this particular path. But it was His plan, and I was on His schedule. There were plenty of bad times, tough times, and there were times when I doubted my faith. More than once I asked, 'Why me?' One day, I was reading in the book of Isaiah, and I came across the passage in chapter 40 where he says, 'Who has measured the Spirit of the LORD, or shown him his counsel, or made him understand, or showed him the way of understanding?' And I thought, 'Why *not* me?' When things got really bad, I would read those verses over and over again, and I found peace. And I kept praying, just like so many of you in this room did. I prayed for God to take away my cancer...and He did.

"Please remember when we have sickness, or when we lose loved ones or our friends, or when terrible things come our way, remember to take time to think and listen and pray. God has a plan for us all—everyone in this room. No matter how bad things are, God has a plan, and He doesn't make mistakes. And I can tell you that through all of this, He never left my side. Sharon and I have been through a lot, and what we've been through has changed me. I see things differently now, and I don't sweat the small stuff. At the end of the day, I know there are two things in my life—two rocks that I can cling to. The first is the Lord. He never fails. And the second is Sharon. I don't know what..."

The words caught in his throat, and tears filled his eyes. No one spoke.

He cleared his throat and said, "So, there you have it. Thanks for your love and prayers, and thanks for listening. We all need to be sure to keep praying and keep believing."

> *Though I walk through the valley of the shadow of death,*
> *I will fear no evil: for thou art with me* (Psalm 23:4 KJV).

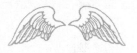

Doxology

While writing this book, we lost our ten-year-old golden retriever, Doxology (Dox). If you've loved and lost a dog, you know the grief and pain this brings. And if you've had a *one-in-a-million* dog—which a lot of us have—you've felt the pain all the more. Dox was a one-in-a-million.

I knew that the moment I first laid eyes on him. I'd driven to a home near Cashiers, North Carolina, to pick him up. He owned me when I first held him in my arms. He was a six-week-old pup, but already an old man. His soft brown, knowing, and piercing eyes took hold of your heart and wouldn't let go. As I drove the four hours back home, he rode in the back of our SUV in a large crate. Each time I glanced in the rearview mirror, our eyes met, and he had me. On at least three or four occasions, I called my wife only to say, "Barbara, this is a special dog." And he was.

For more than seven years, he was the picture of the perfect dog. "The King of Dogs," one of our grandchildren called him. I can't remember him ever being angry or even snarling at a child who rolled over him as if he were a giant stuffed animal. He was perfect, until we noticed a lump under his right eye. It was cancer, and when offered the choices of doing nothing or opting for an aggressive approach, we took the aggressive path. It gave us another three years with him, but it cost Dox his right eye, part of his right jaw, and that cheekbone. You would never know. He was still the calm, loving, perfect dog.

This past Christmas, I noticed a growth in his mouth—another cancer. This time it was melanoma. It was aggressive, and in spite of the best efforts of our veterinarians, we reached a point where there was nothing more to be done. We knew we had only a few months, maybe weeks, and we treasured each remaining moment. We marveled at his steadfast heart, his constant and unwavering love for us and his people, at his bravery. He did everything we asked of him. But we weren't going to allow him to suffer, and on a Monday morning, we said goodbye. It was one of the hardest things Barbara and I had ever done and one of the most painful things we had ever endured. It still is.

One day, when I depart this body and find myself in the presence of the Lord, my time—however it will be measured—will be filled with the praises and the wonder of Jesus. I know that I will once again be able to hug my mother and walk and talk with my father. There are a lot of people I want to see as well: family and friends, grandparents—some of whom I never met on this side. And I will seek out Peter and John and the apostle Paul, as well as other giants of the faith—men and women whose words and deeds have guided and molded my journey and my heart.

We have no idea what heaven will look like—only that it will be perfect. And because of that, I know that one day, when I've experienced the presence and joy of that surrounding host of saints, I will find myself walking with Barbara in a field of lush, green grass, surrounded by gently rising, conifer-cloaked hills.

The words of Jesus will echo through that glade: "Behold, I make all things new." And there will come Dox, charging toward us, his ears flapping in the breeze, his golden hair and majestic tail waving in the wind, and both of his laughing, dancing eyes meeting ours.

> *Praise God, from whom all blessings flow;*
> *Praise Him, all creatures here below;*
> *Praise Him above, ye heav'nly host;*
> *Praise Father, Son, and Holy Ghost.*
> The Doxology

Amen and Amen.

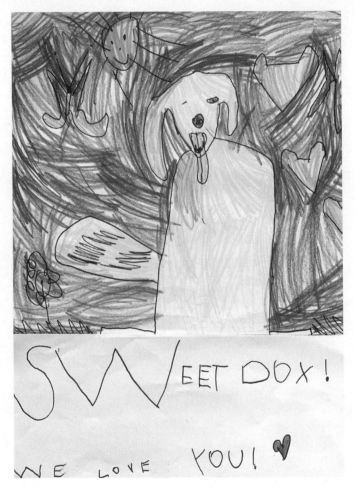

Drawing by our youngest granddaughter, Sadie

About the Author

A physician with more than 30 years of ER experience, **Dr. Robert Lesslie** most recently served as the medical director of a local hospice program. A bestselling author, he has several books to his name (including *Angels in the ER*—over 250,000 copies sold), as well as human interest stories and columns for magazines and newspapers. A fixture in his community, Dr. Lesslie developed two urgent care facilities in South Carolina, a state he and his wife, Barbara, called home for many years.

Other Books By Dr. Robert Lesslie

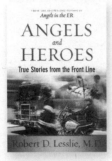

Angels and Heroes

In this unforgettable gathering of inspiring true stories, author of the popular *Angels in the ER,* Dr. Robert Lesslie, shares extraordinary experiences from police, firefighters, and emergency response workers—the men and women who exhibit and witness the grace and strength of angels in the face of danger every day.

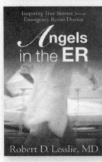

Angels in the ER

Bestselling author Dr. Robert Lesslie offers inspiring true stories of everyday "angels"— friends, nurses, doctors, patients, even strangers—who offer love, help, and support in the midst of trouble. This immensely popular book is a reminder that hope can turn emergencies into opportunities and trials into demonstrations of God's grace.

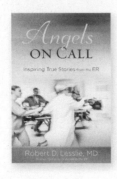

Angels on Call

Fast-paced and inspiring, this collection reveals many nurses, doctors, patients, and friends to be "angels" in their own way. Readers meet patients who choose life despite difficulties, those whose condition demands split-second action, those who triumph over difficulty. An intimate glimpse into the joys and struggles of life.

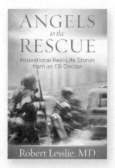

Angels to the Rescue

From bestselling author Robert Lesslie comes a new collection of thrilling inspiration from the emergency room. Join first responders and ER doctors as they encounter life-or-death situations that put their training and faith to the test.

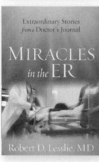

Miracles in the ER

Again and again, bestselling author Robert Lesslie has encountered miracles in the ER during his decades of experience in emergency medicine. In these touching, dramatic, thought-provoking vignettes—all true stories—Dr. Lesslie chronicles real-life stories of life changes, answered prayers, forgiveness, and inner and outer healing where they appeared impossible.